National Children's Bureau Bibliographies

4

The Child with Epilepsy

Rosemary Dinnage

NFER-NELSON

Published by the NFER-NELSON Publishing Company Ltd.,
Darville House, 2 Oxford Road East,
Windsor, Berkshire SL4 1DF, England.

and in the United States of America by

NFER-NELSON, 242 Cherry Street, Philadelphia,
PA 19106–1906.
Tel: (215) 238 0939. Telex: 244489.

First Published 1986

Library of Congress Cataloging in Publication data

Dinnage, Rosemary.
The child with epilepsy.

Includes index.
1. Epilepsy in children – Psychological aspects. 2. Epilepsy in children – Social aspects. 3. Epilepsy in children – Patients – Family relationships. 4. Epilepsy in children – Patients – Education. I. Title. [DNLM: 1. Epilepsy – in infancy & childhood. 2. Epilepsy – psychology. 3. Social Adjustment. WL 385 D585c]
RJ496.E6D56 1986 618.92'853 85–28453
ISBN 0–7005–1024–9

Photoset by David John (Services) Ltd., Maidenhead.

Printed in Great Britain by Henry Ling Ltd., at the Dorset Press, Dorchester, Dorset

ISBN 0–7005–1024–9
Code 8210 02 1

Contents

Acknowledgements

Thanks are due first to the Department of Health and Social Security whose grant made this review possible.

The National Children's Bureau librarians, Ian Vallender and Biddy Cunnell, provided invaluable help in searching for references and obtaining books and photocopies. The British Epilepsy Association was kind enough to supply references.

In particular, thanks are due to Professor Catherine Peckham, Dr Zarrina Kurtz, Mr R.A. Radley and Dr Euan Ross, who read and discussed the manuscript and answered many queries.

Finally, Doria Pilling, whose extensive research review is listed here, is not only responsible for part of the contents but has kindly advised on this updated version.

Introduction

In 1972–73 the National Children's Bureau published a series of concise research review booklets on childhood handicaps. Non-medical studies were summarized, and a brief overview added. In the years since, a great deal of further research and discussion has been published, and the Bureau felt it would be useful to have updated versions. The new booklets, therefore, contain material that was in the originals, together with more recent entries; and the reviews prefacing the annotated bibliographies have been rewritten.

The present booklet is concerned with research on children with epilepsy. Epilepsy is a word that covers a range of disability, from occasional minor fits to frequent, disabling ones that may occur in association with other handicaps such as cerebral palsy. The label 'epileptic' is itself imprecise, as many children grow out of their fits. The fits themselves may be of many different kinds, and there is a considerable literature on classification which is not included here.

What is common to every kind of epilepsy is an electrical malfunction within brain cells. The pattern of the seizure (or fit, or convulsion) is determined by where the brain disturbance is and how it spreads. The malfunction can be caused by a head injury, a tumour, by brain damage during birth, by an illness such as meningitis, by a sensitivity to flickering lights; but in the majority it occurs for no known reason. Anyone can have a seizure, and there are patients who have only one in a lifetime, but to be regarded as 'epilepsy' the fits must be recurrent. The prevalence of uncomplicated epilepsy (not associated with other handicaps) is assessed at between 4 and 5 per 1000.

Roughly, seizures can be classified as 'generalized' or 'partial'. There are two main types of generalized seizure. One is grand mal (also known as tonic-clonic seizures), a total convulsion with unconsciousness, contractions, incontinence of urine, and frothing at the mouth; the other – much more difficult to observe – is petit mal (also known as absences), a blanking out of awareness for a matter of seconds, sometimes frequent in occurrence.

Partial seizures affect only one part of the brain and can be divided into 'simple partial seizures' and 'complex partial seizures'. The former are uncommon, and may affect, for instance, only one limb. 'Complex partial seizures' covers a range of different types of fit, one of the best known of which is the temporal lobe seizure. This may involve a storm of odd emotions or sensations for the patient, and lead to disjointed movements or speech.

These descriptions are, of course, greatly oversimplified; one type of fit may blend into another type, and a patient may have more than one kind. Some fits occur only at night; others only when watching flashing lights.

One other type of fit should be mentioned: febrile convulsions occurring in very young children during an illness with fever. There is controversy as to whether these are connected with true epilepsy in later life, and the subject is not included here. One review article is listed on p.65.

SECTION I

Attitudes to Epilepsy

Epilepsy in particular among illnesses and handicaps has always been regarded with some awe and fear. A grand mal fit – and most people think of 'epilepsy' as grand mal (Harrison and West, 1977) – may indeed be frightening to witness. It is unpredictable, and is associated with loss of control; when demonic possession was believed in, it was a short step to believing that the body was 'taken over' by something unwholesome during a fit. In view of epilepsy's past, therefore, it is not surprising to find that it still carries a stigma which is an added handicap for sufferers. The research would seem to show, however, that public attitudes are improving and even that the stigma is not always as grave as has been feared.

One point in particular must be borne in mind. It will be emphasized again in later sections that 'epilepsy' covers a range of disablement, from the patients able to live a full and normal life to the small proportion whose fits are only part of a cluster of handicaps such as mental retardation and brain damage. When subjects are questioned as part of a research project into public attitudes, they are not asked to distinguish between these groups – and very probably are not clear about the differences.

There are several studies that show up the negative side of attitudes to epilepsy. Among the most pessimistic are Bagley's (1972), who found that a large proportion of his respondents opposed the employment of epileptic people, and that a sample of teenagers placed the epileptic below the cerebral palsied and mentally retarded on questionnaires. As these opinions are more extreme than those found by other researchers, it may be that they are influenced by the number of young and inexperienced people in the sample he questioned. Tringo's (1970) subjects in the USA also rated epilepsy very poorly in a hierarchy of physical and mental handicaps, but again many of his subjects were high-school and college students. An unusual experiment was undertaken by Sands and Zalkind (1972) in the USA: a campaign to educate employers about epilepsy was mounted, but was found to have had no effects on negative attitudes towards employing epileptics.

These studies are not encouraging, but they were all carried out some time ago, and there is evidence that attitudes to epilepsy may be becoming more liberal and informed. Caveness *et al.* (1969) examined answers to polls carried out between 1949 and 1969 and found an encouraging increase in public understanding; a reappraisal five years later

(Caveness *et al.*, 1974) found a further slight increase in enlightened attitudes, and this trend may be continuing.

Certainly more recent studies of attitudes to epilepsy come to rather less pessimistic conclusions. Rather than questioning members of the public, Ryan *et al.* (1980) asked a large group of people with epilepsy in the USA whether they had been stigmatized or discriminated against. 70 per cent said they had not; and while this means, of course, that nearly a third felt they *had,* the result is modestly reassuring. Ryan and his colleagues note that a sense of stigma was more linked with personality factors than with the severity of the epilepsy, which points to the importance of good formative experiences in childhood. A study carried out by Britten *et al.* (1984) focused on the 'visibility' of the child's epilepsy at school and whether it adversely affected behaviour or work; they found that among the children with epilepsy and no other handicaps the obviousness of the disorder was not related to school problems, and conclude that the stigma is not as severe as has been thought.

Two other studies followed the usual method of questioning members of the public about their attitudes. In Australia, nearly half of a group of adults questioned used the word 'normal' in relation to epileptics, 86 per cent believed they should hold jobs like anyone else, and 70 per cent believed the disorder to be controllable (Vinson, 1975); on the other hand, a number of those questioned connected epilepsy with mental illness and crime. Harrison and West (1977) also came up with mixed opinions from adults questioned in this country; those who had actually known people with epilepsy were examined in particular, and while some of them described the epileptic as perfectly normal, others mentioned violence, nervousness, and retardation. These authors make the important point that it is the people with severe epilepsy or multiple problems who are actually visible to the public; no doubt some of those questioned during the study had in fact met epileptic people without ever realizing it.

The attitudes of particular groups have also been looked at. In Australia Beran *et al.* (1981) examined the ideas of some junior doctors and found it regrettable that nearly a third believed epileptics to be below average in their potentialities and work contribution. (It is not clear, however, whether the doctors had the chance to qualify their answers by specifying the great variation among epileptic patients.) The attitude of the schools in this country has been examined by Holdsworth and Whitmore (1974b). They found headteachers seriously under-informed about the epileptic children in their care, but sympathetic in their attitudes. School-fellows too were reported to be generally tolerant and to take the occurrence of a fit in their stride.

This latter finding has some confirmation from Ward and Bower's (1978) study (listed under Section III); the great majority of parents questioned by these authors reported that their children were not victimized by their schoolmates on account of their seizures. Nor did these parents find that rejection by relatives or neighbours was common. If epileptic children do tend to be unpopular at school, findings from the Isle of Wight study (Rutter *et al.*, 1970 (see Sections II and III)) suggest that it is disturbed behaviour rather than the epilepsy itself which is the cause.

An overview of the research on attitudes to epilepsy certainly indicates that adults and children with the disorder have to suffer some degree of stigmatization and misunderstanding, though public attitudes appear to be changing for the better. It would seem that the average person is nervous about fits, uncertain about what epileptic people are capable of accomplishing, and ignorant about the spectrum of disability subsumed in the one word 'epilepsy'. Education of public opinion should be directed towards showing how large a proportion of those suffering from epilepsy lead a normal and productive life. This should go some way to easing the difficulties borne by children suffering from this disorder.

CAVENESS, W.F., MERRITT, H.H., and GALLUP, G.H., JR. (1969) *Epilepsia,* 10, 429–40.

A survey of public attitudes towards epilepsy in 1969 with an indication of trends over the past twenty years

In 1949, 2696 adults in the United States were questioned in a Gallup survey designed to determine the public attitude towards epilepsy. Subjects were selected so that every major group in the population was represented in the same ratio in the samples as in the population. Similar polls were carried out in 1954, 1959, 1964 and 1969. Over the 20 years between 1949 and 1969 attitudes became more favourable towards epilepsy. In each of the five surveys the most favourable attitudes were held by those who were better educated, of higher occupational status, younger and who were from urban rather than rural areas. In 1969 at least 94 per cent of the population had heard of epilepsy. Fewer people in 1969, 9 per cent compared with 24 per cent in 1949, said that they would object to their child attending school or playing with someone who had epilepsy. Only 4 per cent believed epilepsy to be a form of insanity in 1969, compared with 13 per cent in 1949. Over the 20 years there was a 31 per cent increase in the proportion believing that those with epilepsy should be employed as other people are, from 45 per cent in 1949 to 76 per cent in 1969. Even so, 12 per cent still objected to those with epilepsy working.

TRINGO, J.L. (1970) *Journal of Special Education,* 4, 3, 295–306.

The hierarchy of preference toward disability groups

455 subjects from six sample groups, including high school and college students and rehabilitation workers, were asked to indicate the closest relationship they would allow to a person in each of 21 disability groups. Generally the physically disabled were the most acceptable, then the sensorily disabled, while the brain-injured were the least acceptable. Epilepsy was rated more favourably than the other brain injuries, cerebral palsy, mental retardation and mental illness.

BAGLEY, C. (1972) *Epilepsia,* 13, 33–45.

Social prejudice and the adjustment of people with epilepsy

Findings from the present study that more subjects are opposed to employing epileptics than spastics support the author's hypothesis that prejudice against epilepsy is due to fear of sudden loss of physical or emotional control; loss of control in cerebral palsy is consistent and predictable. The questionnaire measuring social attitudes was given to three samples in this country: 574 mainly upper-class teenagers, 211 17- to 19-year-old college students, 104 working and lower-middle-class heads of households. Half of the random sample of adults and a quarter of the college students opposed employing epileptics. In another survey using a social distance scale, 15- to 16-year-olds were found to reject epileptics much more often than either spastics or the mentally ill in relation to work, marriage and housing. It is suggested that prejudice against epileptics plays a significant role in the increased prevalence of behaviour disorders found among people with epilepsy. A review of earlier surveys of attitudes towards epileptics in the United States, Germany, Spain and Britain is included in the article.

SANDS, H. and ZALKIND, S.S. (1972) *Epilepsia,* 13, 87–96.

Effects of an educational campaign to change employer attitudes towards hiring epileptics

In this experimental study an intensive educational campaign in a city in Pennsylvania, which included the use of local radio stations and newspapers, failed to modify the attitudes of executives in a number of large manufacturing companies towards employing epileptics.

Attitude differences between the beginning and end of the experimental period did not differ significantly from differences over this period in a similar Pennsylvanian city in which there was no educational campaign. Fewer than a third of the executives would recommend employing someone with epilepsy.

CAVENESS, W.F., MERRITT, H.H., and GALLUP, G.H. Jr. (1974) *Epilepsia,* 15, 523–6.

A survey of public attitudes towards epilepsy in 1974 with an indication of trends over the past twenty-five years

A Gallup survey on public attitudes towards epilepsy in the United States in 1974 (see Caveness *et al.,* 1969, above) showed a further slight increase in favourable attitudes since 1969.

HOLDSWORTH, L. and WHITMORE, K. (1974b) *Developmental Medicine and Child Neurology,* 16, 6, 759–65.

A study of children with epilepsy attending ordinary schools. 2. Information and attitudes held by their teachers

As part of the study into the progress of 85 children with epilepsy attending ordinary schools, the attitudes of headteachers and the amount of information they possessed were investigated (see also Holdsworth and Whitmore, 1974a, p.35). The headteachers had been informed about the epilepsy of 53 (64 per cent) of the children (by parents, school health service, previous school) and discovered it by chance in a further five children. Even when informed that the child had epilepsy, they were not told of the type of seizure to expect in almost half (41 per cent) of the cases.

Most of the headteachers knew what to do if the child had a fit, but sometimes they only had information from parents, which was occasionally bizarre. The school health service knew that 60 (70 per cent) of the children in the study had epilepsy but had informed the school in only 22 cases, often leaving the school unaware of the child's epilepsy. Nor had the headteachers discussed the children, whose epilepsy they knew about from other sources, with the school health service in the majority of cases. Only two of the 60 headteachers said they would prefer not to admit a child with epilepsy again, but a further teacher said it would depend on the severity of the epilepsy, and five were anxious about coping with a major seizure or the child's management generally. Two said that they were less demanding, and more ready to accept poor work from a child with epilepsy.

Only five teachers thought other pupils had been disturbed by the occurrence of a major fit in a study child at school, though 18 of these children had had their first fit at school. The other children were often sympathetic and tolerant. Many teachers said that the other pupils now 'took it as a matter of course'. It is concluded that social acceptance of a child with epilepsy by teachers and other pupils is welcome, but that teachers often lack information and the lack of discussion between them and school doctors was disturbing.

VINSON, T.
(1975)
Medical Journal of Australia, 2, 663–6.

Towards demythologizing epilepsy

A questionnaire was administered to a representative sample of adults in Sydney, Australia, assessing their attitudes towards epilepsy. Questions about people with other handicaps were included for comparison. 40 per cent described epileptics as 'normal'; but a number of people made associations with emotional problems, mood changes and crime. Asked about schooling for children with epilepsy, 47 per cent said that an ordinary school would be suitable and the rest recommended some kind of special schooling; the former point of view was associated with higher educational status in the respondents.

Only 8.9 per cent said they would be worried if there was an epileptic at their child's school, and 13.4 per cent would be worried if they played at home together. Asked about limitations on epileptics playing sports, 54.2 per cent believed there should be some restriction. 86.2 per cent thought epileptics should be in jobs like anybody else, so long as no danger was involved. About half the sample called the disorder 'mental' and about half 'physical'; 70 per cent believed it was controllable, and 10 per cent curable. 61.5 per cent considered there was an association with mental illness, a much greater number than in the case of the other handicaps.

HANSSON, R.O. and DUFFIELD, B.J. (1976) *Journal of Social Psychology*, 99, 233–40.

Physical attractiveness and the attribution of epilepsy

One hundred college students were shown photographs of young people from the yearbook of a college in another city; the subjects of the photographs had previously been rated for their attractiveness by a panel of students. The hundred subjects were asked to pick out the photograph most likely to be of an epileptic. From the photographs of women, 69 per cent chose an unattractive woman, and from among the men's photographs, 83 per cent chose an unattractive man. They were then rated for several qualities associated with tolerance (empathy, self-esteem, previous acquaintance with an epileptic), but these qualities were not found to have any relation to their choice of photograph. They tended to rationalize their choices of photograph in terms of illness or unhappiness rather than unattractiveness.

HARRISON, R.M. and WEST, P. (1977) *New Society*, 40, 762.

Images of grand mal

114 people in Bristol and Oxford were interviewed to find out what were their 'images of epilepsy'. 'Fits' were generally, but not always, equated with epilepsy. 'Convulsions' were seen as distinct by a significant minority, 28 per cent, being associated with childhood and usually a benign prognosis. Others thought they were quite different, involving vomiting or respiratory problems. The majority of the sample thought of epilepsy as grand mal seizures, involving one or more of the following symptoms: falling to the ground, loss of consciousness, twitching or jerking of the limbs, frothing at the mouth, tongue biting. A quarter associated epilepsy with violence, saying that an 'epileptic' can go berserk.

Some who had known people with epilepsy regarded them as entirely normal, but negative characteristics attributed to 'epileptics' by those with experience included: 'violence' (20 per cent), 'timidity' (20 per cent), 'highly strung' (17 per cent), 'retarded' (17 per cent). The public generally sees the worst side of epilepsy because those with less incapacitating forms of the disorder rarely disclose it. According to the authors, the cure for prejudice against epilepsy is for those with the disorder to reveal and confront it, rather than conceal it.

RYAN, R., KEMPNER, K., and EMLEN, A.C. (1980) *Epilepsia,* 21, 4, 433–44.

The stigma of epilepsy as a self-concept

To study the extent to which people with epilepsy feel stigmatized, a large group of adults with epilepsy in Oregon, USA, were contacted through hospitals, doctors, and through the media. From the total, 445 completed a detailed questionnaire about their health, jobs, and about the attitudes of other people to their disability. Analysis of the answers showed that prejudice was not directly related to the severity of the epilepsy, but was more connected with other factors such as age, education and job experience, and the degree to which the individual *felt* handicapped by his or her disorder. Approximately 70 per cent felt that they had not received unfair treatment because of their epilepsy and were not severely handicapped by it.

BERAN, R.G., JENNINGS, V.R., and READ, T. (1981) *Epilepsia,* 22, 397–406.

Doctors' perspectives of epilepsy

A questionnaire was designed to assess the views of doctors in Adelaide, Australia, on epilepsy. All doctors below consultant status from one hospital were circulated, and out of 111, 69 replied. One part of the questionnaire covered diagnosis and management, and the other part attitudes.

Over half said they were prepared to initiate anticonvulsant treatment; of these, 58 per cent were not prepared to alter the treatment without referral to a specialist. Half the sample said they felt satisfied with their knowledge of epilepsy, but only one-third were satisfied with their knowledge of anticonvulsants. About three-quarters felt that most doctors were not familiar enough with the use of anticonvulsants. 61 per cent had gained their knowledge of epilepsy from undergraduate training, and of these nearly half believed that medical courses give inadequate instruction. 94 per cent had seen a seizure before qualifying.

The doctors were then asked about their attitudes towards employment, driving and social behaviour in relation to epilepsy. Approximately 70 per cent indicated that people with epilepsy contributed as much to society as other people, but that they faced a restricted job market; and 80 to 85 per cent denied that epileptic people need avoid work that is physically or mentally stressful. Over half believed that a driving restriction should be imposed for one to two years after a fit. 30 per cent of the sample felt that epileptic people rated lower than average in intelligence and education, and the same percentage regarded it as unwise for them to have children. The authors argue that the study shows doctors' knowledge about epilepsy and its management to be inadequate, and also point out how regrettable it is that about a third saw epileptic people as below average in their attributes and their contribution to society.

Britten, N., Wadsworth, M.E.J., and Fenwick, P.B.C. (1984) *Journal of Epidemiology and Community Health*, 38, 4, 291–5.

Stigma in patients with early epilepsy: a national longitudinal study

From a longitudinal cohort study of 5362 children, the 46 patients who were identified as having epilepsy were studied. Age of onset of the seizures ranged from babyhood through to adulthood. The main purpose of the research was to see whether the visibility of the handicap was closely correlated with problems at school and work. It was found, first, that poor school achievement was related to early age of onset, and also to complicated cases (those that had other central nervous system disorders as well as epilepsy); uncomplicated cases performed as well at school as their peers. Then each child was rated on an 'index of social visibility' of the disorder, as compiled from teachers' reports on the child at adolescence. 'Visibility' was in fact related to poorer school and after-school performance where the whole group was concerned; but, again, not for the uncomplicated cases, which were the majority. Psychiatric disturbance, however, was higher than average in the group as a whole. The authors' final conclusion is that the actual stigma of epilepsy, as defined by its social visibility, is not in itself as handicapping as has been believed.

Floyd, M. and Lindsay, M. (1984) *Social Work Today*, 15, 43, 14–15.

Portrait of prejudice

It is argued that myths about epilepsy are more harmful to epileptic people than the disorder itself. Some of the mistaken beliefs about it are discussed: that epileptics cannot lead normal working lives, that heredity is a major factor, that fits are catching, that their effects last for hours, that an employee with epilepsy requires special supervision, that he or she will have a high rate of absenteeism, and that there is a particular epileptic personality.

SECTION II

Emotional and Social Adjustment

The evidence for a high rate of emotional disturbance among children with epilepsy is as firmly established as the evidence for an average level of backwardness at school. Once again the unselected sample of the Isle of Wight study provides the most reliable facts: 29 per cent of the epileptic children in the whole of the Isle of Wight were classified as having a psychiatric disorder, as compared to 7 per cent of the rest of the children – that is, four times as many (Rutter *et al.*, 1970).

Other studies are in general agreement. Among epileptic children in the Bristol Child Development Study, nearly a third of the older children had had treatment for emotional problems as compared to only 1 in 25 in the whole of the National Child Development Study, which represents the general child population (Ross and Evans, 1972; Ross, 1974). The method of Mellor *et al.* (1974) was to ask teachers to rate the adjustment of the children in their care, and nearly twice as many of the epileptic children were rated maladjusted as of the other children. Bagley's very detailed study (1971), though admittedly biased towards epileptic children with neurological problems, also found that nearly half had received treatment for psychiatric difficulties.

Is there any particular psychiatric syndrome peculiar to children with epilepsy? Reviews of the research evidence (Scott, 1978; Pilling, 1980 (see Section V, p.62); Reynolds and Trimble, 1981 (see Section V, p.63); Fenton, 1983 (see Section V, p.64)) do not support the old idea of an 'epileptic personality'; in general, epileptic children are disturbed in just the same variety of ways as other children. Bagley (1971) distinguished between the aggressive and the neurotic type of childhood disturbance and found roughly the same proportion of them among disturbed epileptic children as among disturbed non-epileptic children. Mellor *et al.* (1974) mention unhappiness and solitariness as the most notable characteristics of disturbed epileptic children. However, several studies mention restlessness and hyperactivity as being characteristic of children with epilepsy (Mellor *et al.*, 1974; Rutter *et al.*, 1970; Hackney and Taylor, 1976). It seems likely that this at least can be due to subclinical seizures or the brain dysfunction itself; the issues are discussed in Reynolds and Trimble (1981).

There has been much discussion about why children with epilepsy should be prone to emotional maladjustment. There are, of course, some very obvious reasons: a child with a frightening, handicapping, and stigmatizing disability may understandably find life difficult and feel different from his or her contemporaries. There is a suggestion that the epileptic child reacts in particular to a sense of powerlessness; Mathews *et al.* (1982) devised tests measuring self-esteem and 'perception of control' for a small group of epileptic children, and found they had very low scores. In addition, Hartlage *et al.* (1972) and Hoare (1984b) also found that their handicap made epileptic children very dependent.

It is suggested, however, by Rutter *et al.* (1970) that these obvious reasons are not enough to account for epileptic children's high rate of psychiatric disturbance, and they believe that brain dysfunction can be the cause of both handicaps. Pilling (1980), reviewing the literature, argues that asthma is also a frightening and disabling condition, and yet does not produce so much psychiatric handicap. Hoare's (1984a) study would also suggest that neurological dysfunction predisposes to both epilepsy and psychiatric disorder, for newly diagnosed epileptic children were found to be just as disturbed as those who had had the disability for a long time.

Attempts have been made to relate specific types of neurological or epileptic disturbance to specific types of psychiatric disturbance (Bagley, 1971; Stores, 1977; Stores and Piran, 1977; Scott, 1978; Stevens and Hermann, 1981; Hermann, 1982; Whitman *et al.*, 1982). Once again the evidence is complex and draws on medical research which is outside the scope of this review, and the reader is referred to Pilling's (1980) more detailed review and to Reynolds and Trimble's (1981) collection of relevant articles. Reviewing several studies, Stores (1978) isolates three disabling factors: persistent left temporal spike discharge, anticonvulsant drugs, and the fact of boys being generally more at risk than girls. Bagley (1971) found brain damage to be associated with the aggressive, but not the neurotic type of disturbance.

Anticonvulsant drugs may contribute to emotional disorder as well as to learning difficulties (Özdirim *et al.*, 1977 (see Section IV); Hoare, 1984a), but the evidence is difficult to establish. Environmental factors – poverty, bad housing, family pathology – are all of course relevant as well. Bagley (1971) in a long and detailed study examined these factors, and found a clustering of adverse environmental facors in the backgrounds of part of his sample.

All the factors discussed above are undoubtedly related to the high level of emotional disturbance in children with epilepsy, and one must agree with Bagley that they all interact. It does seem probable, in addition, that in a number of children neurological disturbance underlies both the fits and the symptoms of maladjustment. There is, finally, evidence that for some children at any rate the prognosis for adjustment in adult life is better than would have been expected; Lindsay *et al.* (1979a, 1979b, 1979c), when they followed up a very handicapped group of children with temporal lobe epilepsy into adulthood, found 70 per cent to be living normal lives, although a large number had had psychiatric problems in childhood.

RUTTER, M., GRAHAM, P., and YULE, W. (1970) Chapter 12 in *A Neuropsychiatric Study in Childhood.* London: Spastics Society International Medical Publications in association with Heinemann.

The prevalence of psychiatric disorder in neuro-epileptic children

The rate of psychiatric disorder was 29 per cent among children aged 5 to 14, living on the Isle of Wight and identified as having uncomplicated epilepsy (see also p.32 and p.33). This was four times as high as the rate of 7 per cent found among the general population of children on the Isle of Wight, aged 10 to 11. It was also more than twice as high as among children with physical disorders not involving the brain (12 per cent). The rate of psychiatric disorder was higher among children with structural brain damage, but without fits (38 per cent) and even higher among those in whom structural brain damage was accompanied by fits (58 per cent). The diagnosis of psychiatric disorder was arrived at by a psychiatrist, using all the evidence from an interview with the parent, report from the child's class teacher and a psychiatric interview with the child.

The authors ask why the rate of psychiatric disorder is so much higher among children with epilepsy, and other disorders involving the brain. Social prejudice seemed to play only a minor role. Children with epilepsy were reported, by teachers and parents, as being not much liked by other children or 'rather solitary' more often than children with asthma. However, differences between neuro-epileptic children with psychiatric disorders and those without were much greater, suggesting that it may be that the children 'are not much liked' because of their psychiatric disorder, rather than prejudice against them being a cause of the disorder. Social prejudice is also highly unlikely to account for psychiatric disorder being more than twice as high among children with lesions above the brain stem, such as those with cerebral palsy, than among children with lesions below the brain stem, such as those with muscular dystrophy. Low intelligence cannot account for the differences, even though it is known to be associated with psychiatric disorder, for the children with uncomplicated epilepsy had normal intelligence. The authors suggest that the presence of organic brain dysfunction is the main reason for the higher rate of psychiatric disorder among the children with neuro-epileptic disorders.

BAGLEY, C. (1971) London: Routledge & Kegan Paul.

The Social Psychology of the Child with Epilepsy

A detailed study of psychiatric disturbance in children with epilepsy, relating it to type of epilepsy, possible brain damage, social background and family adjustment. Thirteen chapters reviewing the literature on all aspects of the subject are included. The sample consisted of 118 children with epilepsy from a hospital neurological department (average age 14), and their parents. Parents were interviewed at length about the children, and the level of emotional disturbance in each child rated on a number of items on a four-point scale. In addition, 83 epileptic children who were definitely psychiatrically disturbed were compared with disturbed children who were not epileptic.

It was found that nearly half the whole sample was disturbed enough to need the help of child guidance, as compared to 7 per cent in the general child population. There was behaviour disturbance of both the aggressive and the neurotic or anxious type. Difficult environments and parental pathology were related to emotional disturbance, but not frequency of fits or length of time since they started. There were more adverse background factors where there was a near relative with epilepsy. Brain damage was associated with minor fits with motor involvement, with aggressive behaviour disorder, and with hyperactivity. Average IQ was 99.85, and the aggressive children tended to have the lower scores. No firm conclusions could be drawn about the effect of anticonvulsant medication.

Over half of the children's teachers were unaware of their handicap, and communication between hospital and school was inadequate. Teachers tended to underestimate the child's IQ because of retardation in school subjects. In general, adverse environment, family pathology, low intelligence and behaviour disorder tended to cluster together and to reinforce one another.

Hartlage, L.C., Green, J.B., and Offutt, L. (1972) *Epilepsia,* 13, 27–30.

Dependency in epileptic children

Epileptic children were found to be more dependent (Children's Dependency Scale) than children of similar age undergoing tonsillectomy or suffering from cystic fibrosis. Parents of children in the three groups differed in only one of 13 parental attitude factors (Parental Attitude Research Instrument), those of epileptic children most strongly favouring suppression of aggression. None of the parental attitude scores correlated significantly with the dependency scores of the children. Nor did the type or frequency of the seizures, the EEG abnormality or the anticonvulsant medication dosage correlate with dependency in the epileptic children. It is suggested that an explanation for the greater dependence of the epileptic children must be sought in the direct impact of epilepsy or its treatment on the child's psychological development. The 51 epileptic children, average age 11 years 4 months, were randomly selected from a medical out-patients clinic and matched with two other groups of children, tonsillectomy patients and those with cystic fibrosis, of similar age. There were approximately equal numbers of boys and girls in each group and all the children were attending school.

ROSS, E.M. and EVANS, D. (1972) *Epilepsia,* 13, 7–12.

Epilepsy in Bristol secondary school children

Out of 90,000 Bristol children aged 2 to 16 years, 382 were identified as having some form of convulsive disorder (either active at the commencement of the study in 1969 or having required suppressive treatment within the preceding two years). Data were drawn from the medical records of Bristol hospitals and local authorities. A sub-sample, consisting of the 126 secondary school children with epilepsy (aged 11 to 16 years), was studied further by interviewing the parents.

From parents' descriptions of the attacks the great majority of the children, 94, seemed to have had grand mal seizures, while six had petit mal attacks and 11 mixed or indefinite types of attack. Nearly a fifth of the children had had their first attack before they were one year old and well over half before they were five years of age. There appeared to be a high rate of psychiatric attendance among the children in the sample, nearly one-third having attended a hospital child psychiatric department or a local authority child guidance clinic; this was often for the purpose of assessment, however. Two-thirds of the children were supposed to be taking anticonvulsant drugs but 12 out of these 75 children were not taking the medication as prescribed. The activity most restricted on medical advice was riding a bicycle, but only four of the children were considered too handicapped to go swimming. (See also p.16.)

MELLOR, D.H., LOWITT, I., and HALL, D.J. (1974) In: HARRIS, P. and MAWDSLEY, C. (Eds). *Epilepsy.* Edinburgh: Churchill Livingstone, 313–6.

Are epileptic children behaviourally different from other children?

Questionnaires were sent out to 308 teachers in Scottish local authority schools regarding the behaviour of epileptic children and of control children matched for age and sex. Teachers were unaware that the study concerned epilepsy. 295 questionnaires were completed; the significance of the difference between scores of the epileptic child and his or her control was then assessed. It was found that 27 per cent of the epileptic children had a behaviour disorder as compared to 15 per cent of the controls.

The results were then scrutinized to see whether traits characteristic of the 'epileptic personality' emerged. There was no evidence of greater aggression in the epileptic children (in fact, fewer of them were assessed as belligerent), but ten items were more common among them. They were more often assessed as unhappy, unpopular, restless, and having a short attention span (all at a highly significant level); complained of aches and pains, were destructive, bit their nails, were solitary, had speech difficulties, and were disobedient (at a fairly significant level). When the disturbed children from each group were compared, the outstanding characteristics of the disturbed epileptic children were unhappiness and solitariness.

Ross, E.M. (1974) University of Bristol, Doctorate of Medicine thesis.

A Bristol study of secondary school children with epilepsy

Subjects were 110 secondary school children with epilepsy in Bristol (excluding those in mental deficiency hospitals) drawn from those of the 126 in the age group who had been identified as epileptic in the Bristol Child Development Study and who were available for study. Information was obtained from an interview with the parents, a physical examination of the child, and a review of medical records.

In 56 epilepsy was their only major handicap, while 54 had other major physical or psychological disorders – 23 were educationally subnormal, 15 severely mentally retarded and 15 had cerebral palsy. Sixty-seven children were not having seizures in the 12-month period before the study was completed. Twenty-seven out of the 38 still having fits were having grand mal attacks, one was having petit mal on its own, six were having petit mal combined with other forms of fits, and one psychomotor seizures. The prevalence rate was found to be 4.3 per 1000.

Findings do not support the theory that epilepsy is often inherited. Possible perinatal causes were severe asphyxia at birth (three cases), other problems occurring before or at birth (e.g. prolonged labour – six cases), severe jaundice and presumed kernicterus in the first week of life (three cases), some of which might have been prevented by more effective treatment. Five children suffered from congenital disorders which may have been related to their epilepsy. In nine children serious illness after the first week of life, which might have been ameliorated by earlier treatment, are possible causes of the epilepsy. No likely cause for epilepsy was found in 70 of the children.

38 per cent of the epileptic children, compared with 1 per cent of randomly selected Bristol control children, were attending special schools. Only two children were at special 'epilepsy' schools, all the children at special residential schools being placed for reasons other than epilepsy – mainly mental retardation or behaviour problems. About 20 per cent of the epileptic children compared with 7 per cent of the National Child Development Study sample had had more than one month off school in the last year, reasons appearing to be psycho-social rather than due to the fits themselves. As in other studies of epileptic children, a high rate of psychiatric disorder was found.

One in three of the children with epilepsy and no other major handicap had attended the child psychiatric services compared with 1 in 25 in the NCDS sample.

37 per cent of the children were not taking anticonvulsants and did not seem to need any. 18 per cent of the sample appeared to be inappropriately treated, being over- or under-medicated, or in three cases not being seen at a consultant clinic at all, while 15 per cent were not taking the drugs as prescribed. 46 per cent of the sample had been seen at a hospital clinic during the previous year and it was judged that an additional 24 per cent, predominantly multi-handicapped and from working-class homes, would have benefited from attendance. Twenty-five sets of parents complained about the hospital services, the most common complaints being lack of continuity, difficulty of talking to the doctor, and long periods spent waiting. It is suggested that special epilepsy clinics should be set up, and that efforts should be made in each local community to identify all cases and ensure that treatment is adequate. (See also p.15.)

HACKNEY, A. and TAYLOR, D.C. (1976) *Epilepsia*, 17, 275–81.

A teachers' questionnaire description of epileptic children

Four groups of children were studied. Epileptic Group A (30 children who had been in-patients at a children's neuropsychiatric hospital) were compared with Psychiatric Group A (30 child psychiatric in-patients, matched for age, sex and IQ); Epileptic Group B (30 epileptic children who had *not* been in-patients) were compared with School Controls Group B (30 matched normal children from the same schools). The class teachers of these 120 children completed, for each child, the teachers' questionnaire devised by Rutter and Yule and used in the Isle of Wight studies (see pp. 13, 32, 33). The questionnaire is divided into a 'neurotic' sub-score and an 'antisocial' sub-score.

Between the two A groups there were no significant differences; both these in-patient groups had high scores for neurotic and antisocial symptoms. There were, however, significant differences between the Epileptic Group B and Controls Group B (non-handicapped children); and also between the A groups and B groups. The distribution of scores suggested that there were a number of epileptic children who could not be described as psychiatrically disturbed but who were coming to the notice of their teachers with various minor behaviour disorders. In general, there were eight items that characterized the epileptic children: fidgetiness, unpopularity, solitariness, irritability, twitches and mannerisms, unresponsiveness, stuttering, and aggressivity when corrected.

These may all reflect disturbances of motor function or minor seizures, together with the child's natural distress and anger about the handicap.

STORES, G. (1977) In: PENRY, J.K. (Ed) *Epilepsy: proceedings of the eighth international symposium.* New York: Raven Press, 245–9.

Behaviour disturbance and type of epilepsy in children attending ordinary school

Although studies have consistently shown above-average rates of disturbed behaviour among children with epilepsy, few have attempted to investigate whether this is found to apply equally to children with different types of epilepsy. In the present study 70 children with epilepsy who were attending ordinary schools and had had their EEGs recorded at an Oxford hospital were divided into four groups on the basis of their EEG patterns: (a) 3 per second regular spike-and-wave; (b) irregular spike-and-wave; (c) right temporal lobe spike; (d) left temporal lobe spike. The sub-groups were similar in mean age (10 to 11 years) and all contained roughly equal numbers of boys and girls. The behaviour of the children with epilepsy, and of 103 controls, was assessed by means of the Connors' Teacher Rating Scale. Girls with epilepsy differed little from their non-epileptic controls, the only significant difference being that the 3 per second group were more inattentive and over-active. In contrast, boys in all the epileptic sub-groups were more anxious and inattentive, and all except the 3 per second spike-and-wave group were more socially isolated than the non-epileptic boys. The left temporal spike group were also more over-active, making them the most disturbed group.

STORES, G. and PIRAN, N. (1977) *Psychological Medicine,* 8, 441–5.

Dependency of different types in school-children with epilepsy

There is some support for the idea that concern and anxiety about their seizures may make children with epilepsy more dependent on their parents than other children, even those with handicaps. However, there has been no investigation of whether this applies equally to children with various types of epilepsy. The present study investigated dependency in 65 children with epilepsy attending ordinary schools, whose EEG, recorded at an Oxford hospital, consistently showed a single type of abnormality. On the basis of their EEG patterns the children were divided into three sub-groups: (a) generalized seizure discharges; (b) left temporal focal spike; (c) temporal focal spike. In each sub-group the children had a similar average age (10 to 11 years) and there were roughly equal numbers of boys and girls. Dependency was measured on the Self-Administered

Dependency Questionnaire (Berg, 1974), completed by the child's mother, and scores were compared with those of the general population.

Epileptic boys of primary school age had a greater need for close physical emotional contact with their mother and for their mother's presence when they were away from home than boys in the general population. Secondary school age epileptic boys were more in need of practical assistance. Girls with epilepsy were not different from girls in the general population on any type of dependency. Both boys and girls with a left temporal spike had a greater need for close physical emotional contact with the mother than those with a generalized seizure discharge (difference statistically significant) and right temporal spike (difference statistically significant for girls).

SCOTT, D.F.
(1978)
British Journal of Psychiatry, 132, 417–30.

Psychiatric aspects of epilepsy

A discussion of literature up to 1978 on the occurrence and variety of psychiatric disorders in patients with epilepsy. It reviews definition and classification, the relation of epilepsy to intellectual functioning, the incidence of psychiatric disorder with particular reference to personality change, and finally the kinds of neurotic and psychotic disorders encountered in epilepsy. When all epileptic patients are considered together, psychiatric morbidity seems to be high, but there is no specific 'epileptic personality'. There is some evidence of aggressiveness being linked with early onset of epilepsy, particularly in temporal lobe patients; subclinical seizures and consequent confusion may be involved. Depression is the commonest diagnosis for epileptics admitted to psychiatric carc. There is some evidence that patients may have hysterical 'seizures' which mimic genuine ones. The connection between epilepsy and schizophrenia remains confused.

STORES, G.
(1978)
Developmental Medicine and Child Neurology, 20, 4, 502–8.

School-children with epilepsy at risk for learning and behaviour problems

A review of recent research done by Stores and his associates (see pp.18, 35, 37, 40). The evidence suggests that three factors contribute to behaviour problems in children with epilepsy: boys are more disposed to disturbance than girls; a persistent left temporal spike discharge is associated with various symptoms of disturbance; and anti-epileptic drugs, especially phenytoin, are a potential source of serious behaviour disturbance.

LINDSAY, J., OUNSTED, C., and RICHARDS, P. (1979a) *Developmental Medicine and Child Neurology*, 21, 3, 285–98.

Long-term outcome in children with temporal lobe seizures. I. Social outcome and childhood factors

One hundred persons with temporal lobe seizures, first studied as children in 1964, were followed up into adult life. One-third had suffered brain damage, one-third status epilepticus, and one-third had no known cause for the disorder. The patients were divided into four groups: A (independent and seizure-free), B (independent but receiving anticonvulsant medicine), C (dependent), and D (died before 15). There were respectively 33, 32, 30 and 5 in the four groups.

In group A, 55 per cent had an unknown aetiology, 30 per cent had had status epilepticus, and 15 per cent brain insult; most were married and in good employment. In group B, 41 per cent had an unknown aetiology, 25 per cent had status epilepticus, and 34 per cent brain insult; there was a range of good to poor outcomes in employment and marriage; seven of the 32 had successfully undergone lobectomy. In group C, 53 per cent were from the brain injury group and 40 per cent from the status epilepticus group, and only 7 per cent had an unknown aetiology; many had additional handicaps. They were being cared for at home or in institutions. In group D, three of the five children had died of their epilepsy.

Details are also given of the types of brain insult, the outcome of status epilepticus, and the genetic factor in early febrile seizures. Low intelligence, early onset of seizures, grand mal experience, frequency of seizures, hyperkinetic syndrome, and rage attacks were all predictive of poor outcome. The group C patients (at home and in institutions) nearly all derived their handicaps from brain insults which are preventable. The findings indicate a need for skilled review of the requirements of children with limbic seizures, in early years and into adult life.

LINDSAY, J., OUNSTED, C., and RICHARDS, P. (1979b) *Developmental Medicine and Child Neurology*, 21, 4, 433–40.

Long-term outcome in children with temporal lobe seizures. II. Marriage, parenthood and sexual indifference

A further study of the sample of 100 subjects. Here, those who died, and those who were dependent at home or in institutions, were excluded, leaving 66 patients for the study of marriage and sex patterns. Of the 41 men, 17 were married; of the 25 women, 23. Early remission of seizures was strongly linked with marriage; comparing the married men with the unmarried men, it was the only significant factor distinguishing them. Of the 24 unmarried men, at least 14 were found to have a very noticeable absence of sex drive in their lives. Sixty-three children had been born to the 66 subjects, but of these, 41 were the children of the

25 marriageable women and only 22 the children of the 41 marriageable men. The sexual indifference of a number of the men might have been connected with epileptic disruption of hippocampal and amygdaloid function in adolescence.

LINDSAY, J., OUNSTED, C., and RICHARDS, P. (1979c) *Developmental Medicine and Child Neurology,* 21, 5, 630–6.

Long-term outcome in children with temporal lobe seizures. III. Psychiatric aspects in childhood and adult life

Third article in this series on 100 subjects. When the patients were examined as children, a high rate of psychiatric disturbance had been found, as well as disordered homes, mental deficiency, rage outbursts, the hyperkinetic syndrome, and school backwardness. The adult patients were examined for these factors.

Mental deficiency: nearly a quarter of the sample now had verbal IQs below 70; of these, a number were severely retarded or psychotic, and were institutionalized. Hyperkinetic syndrome: 26 children had suffered from this; it proved to be a predictor of poor adult outcome, as only two of the 26 were functioning normally in adulthood. Rage outbursts: this was also a predictor of poor adult outcome, as over half of those with the symptom were psychiatrically disturbed in adulthood. Disordered homes: this factor bore no significant relationship to adult psychiatric problems.

Three psychiatric categories were set up – psychosis, antisocial behaviour, and neurosis – and the adult patients' status examined. Psychosis: 10.3 per cent were overtly psychotic; the condition was associated with a left-sided epileptic focus, severe seizures, and a lack of early remission of seizures. The antisocial group: over 10 per cent of the sample had exhibited seriously antisocial behaviour; this was linked with an epileptic focus contralateral to the preferred hand, severe seizures, and a lack of early remission of seizures. Neurosis: only five patients had been treated for neurotic symptoms. Finally, it is pointed out that while 85 per cent of the patients as children had had psychiatric or learning problems, in adulthood only 30 per cent had the severe problems outlined above – i.e. 70 per cent of the sample were in fact living successful adult lives. It would seem that there is a strong restorative force at work in children who are apparently gravely handicapped.

STEVENS, J.R. and HERMANN, B.P. (1981) *Neurology,* 31, 1127–32.

Temporal lobe epilepsy, psychopathology, and violence: the state of the evidence

A review article with 50 references. The authors examine the studies which have found an association between temporal lobe epilepsy and increased psychopathology, and argue that most of them have been unreliable because they did not include a control group. They conclude that it is brain damage rather than the temporal lobe epilepsy itself which predisposes to psychopathology.

HERMANN, B.P. (1982) *Epilepsia,* 23, 5, 545–54.

Neuropsychological functioning and psychopathology in children with epilepsy

An investigation into the question of what specific factors in epileptic children predispose them to have more behaviour disorders than average. Fifty children from an epilepsy centre in the USA aged 8 to 12 were classified into two groups on the basis of their performance on a battery of neuropsychological tests (motor, tactile, visual, language, memory, etc.). Those with good neuropsychological functioning were then compared with a closely matched group with poor neuropsychological functioning on a checklist of behaviour problems and social competence. The children with poor neuropsychological functioning showed significantly more aggression and general psychopathology, and significantly less social competence, than the other group. Thus a clear link was found between neuropsychological functioning and factors in the child's life such as friends and hobbies, as well as school attainment and behaviour problems.

LEWIS, D.O. PINCUS, J.H., SHANOK, S.S., and GLASER, G.H. (1982) *American Journal of Psychiatry,* 139, 7, 882–7.

Psychomotor epilepsy and violence in a group of incarcerated adolescent boys

Ninety-seven delinquent boys in a correctional school in Connecticut, specially segregated because of their violence, were studied. They were graded 1 to 4 according to how much violence they had demonstrated: in group 1 there were eight boys; in group 2, 11; in group 3, 55; in group 4, 23. Detailed medical histories were compiled, and signs of epileptic illness recorded. 78 per cent of the boys studied had one or more signs characteristic of psychomotor epilepsy. For 74 boys there were EEG records; of these, 25 per cent had an abnormal EEG and/or a history of generalized seizures. A positive correlation was found between number of epileptic signs and degree of violence. Epileptic signs did correlate significantly with hallucinations and paranoia, but not with neurological symptoms. Studying medical records and reports, it seemed that 11 of the 97 boys definitely had seizures, and another seven probably did. The study indicates that there is a high prevalence of psychomotor seizures in the violent delinquent population, and it is important that this is realized.

MATHEWS, W.S., BARABAS, G., and FERRARI, M. (1982) *Epilepsia,* 23, 6, 671–81.

Emotional concomitants of childhood epilepsy

Three matched groups of children in New Jersey were chosen for study: 15 well children, 15 with diabetes, and 15 with epilepsy of various kinds. Any children with associated disabilities were eliminated. An investigator, starting out without knowledge of which group the child belonged to, visited each child's home and administered tests measuring 'perception of control' and self-concept, together with the Draw-a-Person test, which assesses the child's interests and maturity. Then the investigator interviewed the parents at length and got them to complete a test measuring the child's social competence (during this time it became clear which group the child belonged to).

When the test scores were compared, some scores on the 'perception of control' scale showed that the epileptic children were more likely than the others to feel that they lacked control over their lives. Epileptic children also had significantly low self-esteem scores; and they showed a higher level of anxiety than well children on scores derived from the Draw-a-Person test. The parents' reports on social competence confirmed these findings: both the handicapped groups were seen to have problems as compared to the well children, but the items particularly distinguishing epileptic children were lack of initiative, inability to defend themselves, immature behaviour, periods of emotional upset, aggression towards parents, and special problems at school. Ways in which epileptic children's feelings of powerlessness are reinforced are discussed.

WHITMAN, S., HERMANN, B.P., BLACK, R.B., and CHHABRIA, S. (1982) *Psychological Medicine,* 12, 4, 843–53.

Psychopathology and seizure type in children with epilepsy

An attempt to determine whether the presence of a discharging epileptogenic lesion in the temporal lobe is a significant determinant of psychopathology. 153 children from the department of neurology at the University of Illinois were the subjects. Any children attending special schools because of mental handicap were excluded. The cognitive status of the children was assessed by the psychologist, and their behavioural and emotional functioning was also assessed by means of an interview with the child's parents. The children then received a complete neurological evaluation, including an EEG. The subjects were then categorized according to seizure type.

Thirty-five children with temporal lobe epilepsy emerged. The mean aggression scores for the temporal lobe group and the others were compared, as were the Total Behaviour Problems score and the Total Social Competence score. Statistical treatment indicated that no effects of seizure type could be detected on measures of dysfunction, social behaviour, or aggression; that children with temporal lobe seizures do not appear to show increased aggression or decreased competence. However, the factors of male sex and anterior temporal lobe spike activity were associated with behavioural problems, confirming some earlier studies.

HOARE, P. (1984a) *Developmental Medicine and Child Neurology,* 26, 1, 3–13.

The development of psychiatric disorder among schoolchildren with epilepsy

An investigation of psychiatric disorder in four groups of 29 children: one with newly diagnosed epilepsy, one with chronic epilepsy, one with newly diagnosed diabetes, and one with chronic diabetes. The aim of the study was to see whether or not it is the long-continued stress of epilepsy which causes psychiatric disorder, and the diabetic children were used as a comparison group of chronically unwell children. As controls, the next child on the class register of the same sex and age as the index child was chosen. Psychiatric morbidity was assessed by means of the Rutter Scales filled in by parents and teachers.

It was found that there were significant differences in the rate of psychiatric disturbance between the chronic epileptic group and their controls, and – to a lesser extent – between the chronic diabetic group and their controls; and the rate was significantly greater in the chronic epileptic group than in the chronic diabetic group. Between newly diagnosed epileptics and their controls there were significant differences, but not between newly diagnosed diabetics and controls. There was no significant difference between the newly diagnosed and the chronic epileptics.

The epileptic children were then compared on several variables, and it was found that children with focal abnormalities were more disturbed than those with generalized abnormalities, that children with complex partial seizures were more disturbed than those with other categories of epilepsy, that children on the drug phenytoin plus another drug were more disturbed, and that there was a consistent association between severe frequency of fits and psychiatric disturbance. It is concluded that the main findings of the study suggest that, since a high proportion of epileptic children are already disturbed at the time of diagnosis, it is the neurological dysfunction responsible for epilepsy that also predisposes to psychiatric disorder.

HOARE, P. (1984b) *Developmental Medicine and Child Neurology,* 26, 1, 20–24.

Does illness foster dependency? A study of epileptic and diabetic children

Dependency was investigated in a group of newly diagnosed epileptics and a group of chronic epileptics and, for comparison, a group of newly diagnosed and chronic diabetics. A self-administered dependency questionnaire, completed by the child's mother, was used to measure dependency. Children with chronic epilepsy were found to be more dependent than children in the general population, while chronic diabetics did not differ from the general population. Newly diagnosed epileptic children were more dependent than children in the general population on three of the four dependency measures but, again, newly diagnosed diabetic children were not. It is possible that psychiatric disturbance, which was significantly commoner in the two epileptic groups, may also be responsible for inappropriate dependency. Or it is possible (though not likely) that the onset and persistence of epilepsy is more stressful than in diabetes. It is recommended that doctors and teachers help parents to make their epileptic children more independent.

KANGESU, E., MCGOWAN, M.E.L., and EDEH, J. (1984) *Archives of Disease in Childhood,* 59, 1, 45–7.

Management of epilepsy in schools

A consideration of the different community support services for children with epilepsy in an inner-city working-class population. Ninety-two children in south-east London were identified from the handicap register, and clinical details on type of epilepsy, age of onset, seizure frequency, and drug treatment were obtained. Information about community support services was obtained from questionnaires completed by school doctors and from school medical records. 47 per cent of the sample was receiving help from a psychologist, 35 per cent from a social worker, 35 per cent from an education welfare officer, 18 per cent from the psychiatric services, 13 per cent from a speech therapist, and 9 per cent from a physiotherapist. The children in special schools were using more of the support services than the children in ordinary schools.

SECTION III

Educational Attainments

Intellectual Development

Many of the earlier studies investigating the intelligence test scores of children with epilepsy took their samples from those in institutions and clinics and, hardly surprisingly, found them to be inferior to those of control children without the condition. But much previous confusion about the intelligence of epileptic children has been dispelled by the Isle of Wight study (Rutter *et al.*, 1970), which found that the distribution of intelligence in children suffering from epilepsy but no other disorder or injury was roughly similar to that of the general population. This seems to be the first study which has obtained an unselected sample of epileptic children, all those between the ages of 5 and 14 living on the Isle of Wight who had had a fit within the past 12 months or had been on anticonvulsant medication during that period. The average intelligence test score of the epileptic children without other disorder was 102, only slightly lower than that found in another part of the Isle of Wight study for a randomly selected sample of 10- to 12-year-olds, 111.

Other studies have come up with lower average IQs than this for epileptic children, but all have had some bias towards including children with severe or complicated epilepsy. This has lowered the average group score, as such children may certainly suffer from retardation. On a test of reasoning ability, boys with epilepsy attending ordinary schools in Scotland had significantly lower scores than their classmates, for example (Mellor and Lowitt, 1977). However, it is stated that the sample was identified through hospital and other records, and perhaps this led to a bias towards the more severely affected children.

In another British study (Bagley, 1971 (see Section II)) children came from among those attending the neurological department of a London hospital, and so the sample is likely to be biased by children with neurological abnormalities or uncontrollable fits. For this sample the average intelligence score was found to be virtually the same as that for the general population but the curve for intelligence was skewed to the left – that is, there were more cases with low IQ than would be expected in the normal population.

In an American study (Needham *et al.*, 1969) subjects were obtained from those attending welfare and private-practice clinics. Again, this could have biased the sample towards those with greater problems; and probably partly at least accounts for the fact that the average IQ of the epileptic children was slightly lower than that of their siblings, although still near average.

In the Isle of Wight study, children with uncomplicated epilepsy made up about three-quarters of the total number of epileptic children (22 out of 86 had some structural brain disorder), and there remains the question of the more handicapped one-quarter. No separate information is given about the intelligence test scores of the epileptic children with structural brain disorder, but it is available for the group with structural brain damage as a whole. Over half the children with cerebral palsy and 70 per cent of those with other brain disorders showed mental retardation (IQ 70 and below), while the respective figures for severe mental retardation (IQ 50 or below) were 36 per cent and 55 per cent respectively. But although there is undoubtedly a strong connection between brain damage and low intelligence, by no means all epileptic children with brain damage have low intelligence; in Bagley's (1971) study there were a number of children in the upper ranges of intelligence who had possible brain damage, though none with clinically identifiable conditions such as cerebral palsy.

There is one other study which appears to conflict with the findings of the Isle of Wight research; a survey of children under 16 with epilepsy in a region of Finland found that over half of them were to some extent retarded (Sillinpaa, 1973). The sample, though, was not completely unselected as in the study by Rutter and his colleagues. It seems probable that the sample was again biased towards children with handicaps additional to epilepsy, but information is not provided in terms which makes possible a comparison between the two studies.

It seems clear that the large proportion of epileptic children who have epilepsy alone, uncomplicated by other handicaps, have intelligence within the normal range. Whether they have a slight excess of scores at the lower end of the normal range, or whether the samples in most of the studies was slightly biased, cannot be determined from the evidence available.

Do these findings mean that epilepsy itself has no adverse effects on intellectual development, though an organic insult of some sort to the brain may both cause retardation and also predispose the child towards epilepsy? Generally this does seem to be the position. Recurrent seizures do not appear to produce deterioration in subjects with normal intelligence and no clinical evidence of neurological abnormalities.

This picture needs some final qualification, however. Bourgeois *et al.* (1983) found that when a group of epileptic children were given intelligence tests over a period of years, a small group of about 10 per cent did show a gradual decline. The two factors distinguishing the group were a high incidence of anticonvulsant drugs in the toxic range, and early onset of seizures. Specific types of childhood epilepsy have been distinguished which start early and are associated with retardation; the medical evidence is complex and has been reviewed by Pilling, 1980 (see Section V). Status epilepticus, a seizure or series of seizures lasting over half an hour, also has a poor prognosis. These conditions, however, affect only a small minority of children with epilepsy.

Educational Achievement

The outcome of research on epileptic children's school achievement is somewhat less favourable than that on intelligence, for all studies suggest that on average they fall behind the standard that would be expected for their age and intelligence. There are various possible reasons for this, which are discussed in the research literature. There is a suggestion, though, that they tend to catch up in later youth, when seizures may be outgrown (Ross *et al.*, 1980; Lindsay *et al.*, 1979b (see Section II)).

Two-thirds of the children with epilepsy in the National Child Development Study, a representative sample of children throughout Great Britain, were at ordinary schools (Ross and West, 1977; Ross *et al.*, 1980). (Epileptic children in special schools are discussed separately below.) At seven, considerably more (50 per cent) of the epileptic children were graded as poor readers than of the other children (29 per cent). At 11 they were still not doing as well as the non-epileptic children, with low scores in both reading and maths (Ross and West, 1977).

These findings are backed up by those of the Isle of Wight study, which found that 18 per cent of the children with uncomplicated epilepsy were retarded in reading as compared with only 7 per cent of the control children. In another study of epileptic children attending ordinary schools in this country (Holdsworth and Whitmore, 1974a) the criteria for school progress were not definite and there was no control group, but it again appears that a high proportion of the children with epilepsy were having difficulties at school. The most disturbing report is that of Stedman *et al.* (1982); they found that among epileptic children attending ordinary schools in the Oxford region, only 15 per cent could be considered as making fairly satisfactory school progress, and nearly half were more than two years behind in reading, spelling or arithmetic. The sample may not be free of bias towards the more handicapped children, however.

Various reasons have been put forward as to why epileptic children should experience learning difficulties even when they are of adequate intelligence. In an attempt to find out whether the difficulties are due to specific intellectual deficits associated with the epilepsy, some studies have been made relating performance to various types of seizure and EEG pattern. The evidence is complex and has been summarized by Pilling (1980). It seems at any rate that boys tend to have more learning difficulties than girls and that left temporal involvement may be especially handicapping (Stores and Hart, 1976; Stores, 1978 (see Section II)).

The question also arises as to whether some epileptic children's attentiveness in class is disrupted by subclinical seizures which go unnoticed; again, this is a question which goes beyond the limits of this book and which has been assessed by Stores (1973) and Pilling (1980). Stores points out that 'inattentiveness' – a word that tends to be used of epileptic children in school – is a complex thing and that attention involves various cognitive skills. In two studies (Stores and Hart, 1976; Stores, 1977) he tested several aspects of learning and attention in epileptic schoolchildren and related them to EEG patterns. It seems clear that the possibility of disruption of learning by subclinical seizures cannot be ruled out.

Two other obvious factors that may impair school achievement are maladjustment and absence from school. Evidence about school absence is conflicting, Ross, 1974 (see Section II) reporting a rather high rate of absenteeism and the Isle of Wight findings suggesting the contrary (Rutter *et al.*, 1970). Maladjustment, however, is certainly – and understandably – higher than average in children with the handicap of epilepsy (see Section on 'Emotional and Social Adjustment'); and this is very likely to disrupt good progress at school.

One other important factor relevant to epileptic children's school work is that most are taking anticonvulsant drugs, which may have side-effects leading to poor concentration. The literature on anticonvulsant medication is enormous, and again the reader is referred to Pilling's (1980) review. There is no doubt, at any rate, that the perfect drug that controls seizures without any impairing side-effects has yet to be found. Stores (1975) argues that the subject urgently needs more careful research. All the above factors, therefore, are likely to be relevant to educational retardation among epileptic children in ordinary schools.

There remain the children in special schools. Ross (1974) in the Bristol Child Development Study identified 38 per cent of his sample of epileptic children as attending special schools, and Ross *et al.* (1980) in the National Child Development Study found roughly the same proportion. They attended a range of types of special schools and very few were in schools for children with epilepsy, most being multi-handicapped children suffering predominantly from mental retardation. Kurtz (1983) has made a survey of the six special schools for epileptics in England and Wales, and reports that only 5 per cent of the children in them had no handicap beyond epilepsy. Children were very often placed in these residential schools because of a combination of family problems and multiple medical handicaps. Only about a quarter who had left these schools were in employment at follow-up two to five years later.

Finally, a few studies have been listed which give indications of the general course and life performance of unselected groups of epileptic people (Harrison and Taylor, 1976; Lindsay *et al.*, 1979a, 1979b, 1979c; Goodridge and Shorvon, 1983; Okuma and Kumashiro, 1981). In general they show that averages for intellectual and social development among epileptic people are misleading, as there is a range that runs from the minority who have problems throughout life to the majority that achieve well.

NEEDHAM, W.E. *et al.* (1969) *Journal of the American Medical Association,* 207, 8, 1497–1501.

Intelligence and EEG studies in families with idiopathic epilepsy

There is much confusion in the literature over the intelligence of those who suffer from idiopathic epilepsy, i.e. recurrent seizures without a known structural or metabolic basis. The present study investigated the relationship between intelligence and idiopathic epilepsy. The 73 subjects consisted of those with 'petit mal' (typical absences) and those with 'focal idiopathic epilepsy', in whom some other member of the family had a similar epileptoid EEG abnormality. The subjects, and their parents and siblings, were tested by a psychologist on a standard intelligence test according to age, and an EEG recording was taken.

On all the tests used the mean IQs of the subjects with epilepsy were within the average (90–109) or low average (80–90) ranges, and within one standard deviation of the established means of the tests. Generally, on all the tests the subjects with epilepsy had lower scores than their non-epileptic relatives. The exception was that the children did not differ from their young relatives on the verbal scale of the Wechsler. The IQ scores of the non-epileptic relatives with epileptoid abnormalities were little different from those of the relatives who had normal EEGs. 70 per cent of the subjects with epilepsy scored below the median IQ of their close relatives (all tests combined). A greater percentage of subjects with epilepsy than of the standardization populations had scores in the lower categories of the IQ ranges (79 or below) in each of the tests.

It is suggested that the findings of the study reconcile the contradictory views on the intelligence of those with idiopathic epilepsy. As a group they have reduced intellectual functioning, but the majority have average or near-average scores on standardized tests. And in a third of their families those with epilepsy have IQs above the median of their near relatives.

RUTTER, M., GRAHAM, P., and YULE, W. (1970) Chapter 8 in *A Neuropsychiatric Study in Childhood.* London: Spastics Society International Medical Publications in association with Heinemann, 124–32.

Epileptic disorders

All school age children suffering from epilepsy on the Isle of Wight were identified on the basis of school medical and hospital records, an interview with the parents and a neurological examination. Epilepsy was defined as a condition in which there had been at least one overt fit since the age of five and in which the child had had an overt fit or had been taking anticonvulsant medication during the preceding 12 months.

Eighty-six children were diagnosed as epileptic. Prevalence of epilepsy in the 5- to 14-year-old population was found to be 7.2 per 1000. The rate of 'uncomplicated' epilepsy (unassociated with any other known brain disease, disorder or injury) was 5.4 per 1000, while the rate of epilepsy associated with cerebral palsy or some other structural brain disorder was 1.8 per 1000. Half of all the children with epilepsy had only major attacks. 5 per cent of those with uncomplicated epilepsy had petit mal alone, and 16 per cent in association with other types of fit; none of those with a structural brain disorder had petit mal alone but in 5 per cent it occurred in association with other types of fit.

About a fifth of the children had minor attacks only (i.e. all types of fit other than major attacks or petit mal) and 15 per cent in association with major fits. Eight (13 per cent) of the children with uncomplicated epilepsy and three (13 per cent) of those with a structural brain disorder had psychomotor fits, in six of the children these being the only type of fit while the others also had major seizures. Four children (6 per cent) had myoclonic fits. Fourteen (16 per cent) of the epileptic children, 12 (19 per cent) of those with a structural brain disorder, had fits with a focal motor component. In most children these fits began focally and then spread to the other side ending in unconsciousness and general convulsions.

In the majority of cases the fits were well controlled, a third of the children not having had a fit for a year. Two-thirds of those who had major attacks had not had one in the previous year, 13 per cent had only one and 8 per cent had had more than ten fits in the year. Of those with minor attacks 76 per cent had had no attacks during the previous year, and only 11 per cent more than ten attacks. The frequency of attacks was similar for children with uncomplicated epilepsy and those with structural brain disorder.

10 per cent of the children were not taking regular anticonvulsant medication, mainly because the parents did not realize the need for this. (Over half of the children were taking phenobarbitone, and an additional 25 per cent in combination with another drug.) Onset of epilepsy was earlier in those with structural brain disorder, the first attack occurring before the age

of two in almost half of these children. Onset occurred between the ages of two and eight in two-thirds of those with uncomplicated epilepsy, being particularly common between the ages of five and eight. All except four children had seen their family doctor about their epilepsy and only 16 per cent had not attended hospital for this, though referrals were often delayed for some time.

RUTTER, M., GRAHAM, P., and YULE, W. (1970) Chapter 9 in *A Neuropsychiatric Study in Childhood.* London: Spastics Society International Medical Publications in association with Heinemann, 133–49.

Intellectual and educational aspects of neuro-epileptic disorders

Eighty-six children between the ages of five and 14 living on the Isle of Wight were identified as having epilepsy, 64 of them having uncomplicated epilepsy (the fits were not associated with any other known brain disorder, disease or injury). (See also pp. 13, 32.) The IQ (Wechsler) of the children with uncomplicated epilepsy was roughly normal. There was a tendency (not reaching statistical significance) for the average verbal IQ to exceed the average performance IQ. Half of the children with uncomplicated epilepsy were reading adequately, but 18 per cent (of the 50 over the age of eight) were at least two years retarded in reading comprehension (in relation to their age and IQ score). Significantly more of the children with uncomplicated epilepsy than of the random control group were retarded in reading by more than two years. School absence is a possible reason for poor school attainment but the children with uncomplicated epilepsy were absent from school to an only slightly greater extent than the controls (37 and 34 absences respectively).

ROSS, E.M. (1973) *Proceedings of the Royal Society of Medicine,* 66, 7, 701–4 (Section on Epidemiology and Preventive Medicine, 31–4).

Convulsive disorders in British children

In the National Children's Bureau study of all children born in the week 3 to 9 March 1958, 21 per 1000 were found to have suffered from febrile convulsions alone and 4.1 per 1000 from afebrile seizures. Only 2 per 1000 children had a fit between the ages of 10 and 13. Epilepsy was well-controlled in most of the children, only 1 in 3000 having a seizure disorder resistant to treatment. Slightly more boys than girls suffered from both febrile and afebrile convulsions but children from all social classes were equally affected. A higher proportion of afebrile children than controls had weighed under 2500g. at birth and maternal bleeding before 28 weeks was more common among them, but there was no relationship with any other perinatal factors. At seven years of age children with afebrile seizures attending ordinary schools tended to do worse than controls on scholastic tests. 50 per cent were graded as poor readers compared with 29 per cent of the controls, and their performance in copying designs was particularly poor. Children who had febrile convulsions alone did not differ in educational performance from those who had never had fits. (See also p.39.)

SILLINPAA, M. (1973) *Acta Paediatrica Scandinavica,* Supplement 237.

Medico-social prognosis of children with epilepsy. Epidemiological study and analysis of 245 patients

A study of all (245) children under the age of 16 with recurrent epileptic seizures living in the catchment area of the Turku University Central Hospital in Finland, who had been hospitalized for seizures (routine policy in the area) during the period 1961–4. Subjects were followed up for an average period of ten years, at the end of which detailed data on previous history were collected, neurological and other investigations made, and psychological tests administered.

69 per cent of the subjects had one type of epilepsy only, 27 per cent two types and the rest three or more types. Grand mal (tonic-clonic seizures) was the commonest type of epilepsy, occurring in 54 per cent (131) of subjects, as the only form of epilepsy in 79 and in combination with other types in the rest. Psychomotor seizures (complex partial seizures) were the second commonest type occurring in 47 per cent (114) of subjects, in 55 as the sole type of epilepsy. The third commonest type of epilepsy were secondarily generalized partial seizures. Petit mal, partial cortical (focal) epilepsy, infantile spasms, and akinetic-myoclonic epilepsy each occurred in about 5 per cent of the subjects, often in combination with other types. In subjects with early onset of epilepsy all types occurred but psychomotor seizures had their maximum frequency of onset at this stage.

47 per cent of subjects had had attacks more than once a week when they were at their maximum frequency while 8 per cent had not had them more often than once a year. Status epilepticus had occurred at least once in 24 per cent of subjects. Final remission from seizures for more than seven years occurred in 27 per cent (66) subjects. A good prognosis for freedom from seizures was significantly related to normal gross motor, fine motor development and mental state. It was not related to the adequacy of treatment received. No particular type of fit was significantly correlated to a long remission period, but seizure types occurring in isolation were more favourable than combinations of seizures.

Intelligence level was normal (IQ 86 or above) in 47 per cent of subjects, 34 per cent being severely mentally retarded (IQ 51 or below). Intelligence level was highly significantly related to an organic aetiology. 45 per cent of the subjects in the sample who were over the age of 16 were employed, 30.7 per cent were still at school or at college, and 19.8 per cent were unoccupied. Neurotic symptoms occurred in 55 per cent of the sample, psychoneurotic in 30 per cent, psychotic in 11 per cent and hyperkinetic in 33.5 per cent. Definite or probable neurological abnormalities were found to be present in 77 per cent of those with psychopathological disturbances. 44 per cent of the sample were personally independent (able to carry out all the same activities as healthy peers of the same age), and 23 per cent were entirely dependent. Subjects with normal intelligence had a 44 per cent chance of remaining free from seizures for seven years, while the profoundly mentally retarded (IQ 20 or below) had only a 7 per cent chance. 25 per cent of those with normal intelligence could not expect a remission of this length. However, good school performance (in those able to attend school), employment and behavioural disturbances were not correlated with seven years' remission from seizures.

STORES, G.
(1973)
Developmental Medicine and Child Neurology,
15, 376–82.

Studies of attention and seizure disorders

A discussion of 'inattentiveness' in epileptic schoolchildren and a review of relevant work up to the time of writing. The effects of anticonvulsant drugs, subclinical seizures and mental subnormality are considered, as well as types of EEG abnormality, and the influence of psychological factors. Attention and inattention are complex concepts which need clarification, and tests of attention in epileptic children must be carefully designed.

HOLDSWORTH, L. and WHITMORE, K.
(1974a)
Developmental Medicine and Child Neurology,
16, 6, 746–58.

A study of children with epilepsy attending ordinary schools. 1. Their seizure patterns, progress and behaviour in school

A study designed to examine how children with epilepsy fared in ordinary schools, and how they were regarded by their teachers. The study was carried out in one local authority, the names of the children being supplied from the school health service register of handicapped children. Eighty-five children who had had a seizure in the previous 12 months, or were on anticonvulsive therapy during this period were taken as subjects.

Seventy-three children had major fits, but 15 of them also experienced other types of seizures. Twelve (14 per cent) of the children had additional handicaps, two having physical disorders, five being mentally retarded (IQ below 70), and two having speech defects. The progress at school of 64 of the children was graded according to their headteacher's opinion (those below the age of six and one or two others being omitted). Twenty (31 per cent) of the children were maintaining an average to superior performance (group A); 34 (53 per cent) were below-average (group B); and ten (16 per cent) had fallen seriously behind (group C). Thirty-six children (42 per cent of the 85) were described by teachers as inattentive. Eighteen (21 per cent) were considered to be noticeably deviant in their behaviour, 14 being troublesome and aggressive, four isolated or withdrawn. More of those who were failing (groups B and C) were boys. Frequent fits were not more likely among those who were failing. More children with major epilepsy were failing, but almost two-thirds in the group making good progress at school did, in fact, suffer from major seizures.

Nearly all the children with behaviour problems were educationally backward, but only a quarter of the educationally backward had behaviour disorders, suggesting that behaviour problems are not commonly a causal factor. The frequency of fits seemed very important in relation to behaviour disorders, unlike educational failure. There was a high rate of inattentiveness in both the educationally retarded and behaviour disordered groups. The inattentiveness might be associated with subclinical paroxysms occurring between seizures; or anti-epileptic drugs might be causing side-effects.

Medical care and specialist help for these children seemed to be inadequate. Over a half were having more than one seizure a year, and one in six had seizures once a month or more often. A third of the children who had fallen most seriously behind had not been referred to an educational psychologist, and two-thirds with behaviour problems had not been referred for psychiatric help. Nor was there evidence of close cooperation between doctors, psychologists and teachers in the 32 children with frequent seizures, serious educational retardation and behaviour problems.

HARRISON, R.M. and TAYLOR, D.C. (1976) *Lancet*, May 1, 948–51.

Childhood seizures: a 25-year follow-up

A follow-up of 179 epileptic people from a large sample of children originally studied between 1948 and 1953. The original sample had been an unselected one including every kind of case from complicated epilepsy to simple febrile convulsions. The present sample was traced and then interviewed for one to three hours about aspects of their present life.

10 per cent were found to have died, most of them before the age of ten. Another 10 per cent were in institutions, and 6 per cent lived at home without employment. Of the survivors, a quarter continued to have seizures; of these patients who were

still having seizures, only half were self-supporting in the community, the rest being among the institutionalized and unemployed. Of all the survivors, 4 to 10 per cent had been in special education, 19 per cent had reached 'O' level standard, 10 per cent 'A' level standard, and 6 per cent degree-level qualification. Those with continuing epilepsy, however, had reached much lower standards when considered separately. The unemployed nearly all came from the group who remained at home as invalids; among the employed, those whose epilepsy had remitted were in much better jobs than those who continued to have seizures.

The authors argue that in spite of improvements in care and management since the time when these subjects were children, epilepsy's frightening reputation has some justification. Though about two-thirds of subjects were leading normal lives, the one-third who had died or were in institutions must also be remembered – even though their epilepsy may have been incidental to other handicaps.

STORES, G. and HART, J. (1976) *Developmental Medicine and Child Neurology*, 18, 705–16.

Reading skills of children with generalized or focal epilepsy attending ordinary school

Previous research has suggested that children with a certain electrographic type of epilepsy – with recurrent bursts of generalized seizure discharge – may be particularly disadvantaged at school because of inattentiveness. In the present study 17 epileptic children attending Oxfordshire schools, aged 7 to 14 years, who consistently showed this type of EEG were compared on reading achievements with 17 epileptic children matched for age and sex who had persistent focal spike abnormalities in their EEGs. Each epileptic child was also matched with a non-epileptic child in the same school class, of the same sex. Each child's reading achievement was assessed by comparing his or her actual scores on the Neale Analysis of Reading Ability with scores expected for a child of the same age and intelligence.

In terms of mean difference between their actual and predicted reading scores the generalized group did not differ from their controls but the focal group did perform worse than their controls (the difference reached statistical significance on reading accuracy). In the generalized group it was found that children with numerous clinical absence attacks performed no worse than those with relatively infrequent absence attacks. The poorer performance of the focal group children could not be accounted for by school absence or behaviour disturbance. Children with a left hemisphere spike, though, did have poorer reading scores than those with a right hemisphere focus, and most of these children were boys. Epileptic boys (irrespective of EEG type) had significantly worse reading scores than epileptic girls. Also most of the children in the focal group had been taking phenytoin, and children who had been prescribed this drug for at least two years (whatever their EEG type) had poorer reading scores than those who had been prescribed other drugs. In contrast to previous findings, the evidence from this study does not show that children with generalized seizure discharge are especially educationally disadvantaged. It suggests that educational failure in epileptic children is the outcome of a combination of factors.

MELLOR, D.H. and LOWITT, I. (1977) In: PENRY, J.K. (Ed) *Epilepsy: the eighth international symposium*. New York: Raven Press, 291–4.

A study of intellectual function in children with epilepsy attending ordinary schools

Children aged 7 to 15, diagnosed as having epilepsy, and attending ordinary schools in the north-eastern region of Scotland were identified through hospital and other records. 216 of these children with epilepsy were matched with the classmate nearest to them in age and of the same sex, and their scores on the Moray House Test (a test of reasoning ability taken routinely in Scotland at 9 or 11) were compared. Significantly more of the boys with epilepsy, but not the girls, had low scores. This remained so when the six children with symptomatic epilepsy were excluded. Behaviour disorder (as assessed by the Rutter teacher questionnaire) was related to lower Moray House scores in both the children with epilepsy and the controls. The authors suggest that the study findings support the view that children with 'non-organic' epilepsy usually have intellectual abilities within the normal range but there is a tendency for the lower end of the normal range to be over-represented.

ÖZDIRIM, E., RENDA, Y., and EPIR, S. (1977) In: MEINARDI, H. and ROWAN, A.J. (Eds) *Advances in Epileptology*. Amsterdam: Swets and Zeitlinger, 120–3.

Effects of phenobarbitol and phenytoin on the behaviour of epileptic children

The present study used five psychological tests to measure aspects of cognitive, perceptual and adaptive functioning. The subjects were 63 children diagnosed as epileptic, seen at the neurology out-patient department of a children's hospital in Turkey, who had not previously been taking anticonvulsants. The subjects were randomly assigned to one of three treatment groups: placebo, phenobarbitone or phenytoin. The three groups did not differ initially in age, sex, educational level, educational level of parents, or aetiology of epilepsy. Subjects were administered the five tests before the beginning of treatment and three months after it started.

On the Goodenough–Harris Draw-a-Man and Draw-a-Woman tests the average score of the placebo group increased significantly on the second testing, that for the phenytoin group showed a non-significant increase, but that of the phenobarbitone group did not change. All three groups showed increases in their average scores on the Turkish adaptation of the Peabody Picture Vocabulary test. On a Problem Behaviour Rating scale (developed at the clinic) the placebo group showed no change on re-test, but the phenobarbitone group showed an increase, and the phenytoin a non-significant decrease, in undesirable behaviour. None of the groups showed any changes in adaptive behaviour (Vineland Social Maturity Scale) or perceptual–motor functioning (Bender Gestalt). The results indicate that phenobarbitone has an adverse effect on behaviour.

Ross, E.M. and West, P.B. (1977) In: Meinardi, H. and Rowan, A.J. (Eds) *Advances in Epileptology*. Amsterdam: Swets and Zeitlinger, 34–7.

Achievements and problems of British eleven year olds with epilepsy

The behaviour and educational achievements at 11 of the 64 children with definite epilepsy in the National Child Development Study sample (all children born in England, Scotland and Wales during the week 3 to 9 March 1958) were compared with those of the rest of the sample. 67 per cent of the children had tonic-clonic (grand mal) seizures, on their own or combined with typical absences (petit mal). 21 per cent of the children with epilepsy had seen a psychiatrist, compared with 3 per cent of the non-epileptic children. Parents of the children with epilepsy were three times as likely to be considered over-concerned as parents of controls. Two-thirds of the epileptic children were attending ordinary schools, compared with 93.5 per cent of the controls. Of the 21 epileptic children ascertained as in need of special education, epilepsy was the major reason in seven of them. The other children were ascertained on account of educational backwardness (6), severe retardation (3), cerebral palsy (2), behaviour problems (3) and other problems (3). Both the epileptic children at special schools (23 per cent) and at ordinary schools (13 per cent) were much more likely to have missed at least a month's school in their eleventh year than the other children (6 per cent). More of the epileptic children at ordinary schools (46 per cent) than of the controls (30 per cent) had low reading, and maths (40 per cent and 31 per cent respectively) scores. However, on the 'copying designs' test, supposed to measure perceptual–motor ability, the epileptic children performed as well as the non-epileptic. (See also p.33.)

STORES, G. (1977) In: MEINARDI, H. and ROWAN, A.J. (Eds) *Advances in Epileptology*. Amsterdam: Swets and Zeitlinger.

Sex-related differences in 'attentiveness' in children with epilepsy attending ordinary schools

Children with epilepsy are often described as 'inattentive' by teachers but it is not certain what is meant by this or whether 'inattentiveness' occurs equally often among all groups of children with epilepsy. In this study 71 children with epilepsy (36 boys, 35 girls) attending ordinary schools were compared on five measures of attentiveness with 35 non-epileptic children: (1) teachers' ratings of inattentiveness; (2) Werry–Weiss–Peters (WWP) Activity Scale completed by parents and teachers who assessed the child's degree of activity in various everyday situations; (3) Continuous Performance Test (CPT) – the child listened for 16 minutes to a tape of random letters and had to detect numbers which periodically replaced the letters; (4) Visual Scanning test – the child was asked to scan quickly randomized letters and cross out one specified letter each time it occurred; (5) Distractibility test – as (4), but against a background of noise.

The boys with epilepsy were significantly more inattentive than the non-epileptic boys, as measured by teachers' ratings of activity, the second half of the CPT (suggesting a difficulty in sustained attention) and the Visual Scanning test. The girls with epilepsy did not differ from their non-epileptic counterparts. In contrast to the control children, noise in the Distractibility test produced an improved performance in those with epilepsy. When the children with epilepsy were divided into sub-groups on the basis of their EEG patterns, those with the 3 per second regular spike-and-wave pattern had better scores on the second half of the CPT than those with generalized, irregular spike-and-wave or right temporal spikes, and better scores on the Distractibility test than those with either right or left temporal spikes. Some correlation was found between the various measures of attentiveness, with the exception of the teachers' ratings, making the interpretation of these difficult.

CAMFIELD, C.S., CHAPLIN, S., DOYLE, A.B., SHAPIRO, S.H., CUMMINGS, C., and CAMFIELD, P.R. (1979) *Journal of Pediatrics,* 95, 361–5.

Side effects of phenobarbital in toddlers: behavioural and cognitive aspects

Despite its widespread use as an anticonvulsant, and reports of undesirable behaviour changes, there have been remarkably few attempts to investigate the cognitive and behavioural effects of phenobarbitone in children. Subjects in the present study were toddlers taking part in a double-blind study of the efficacy of phenobarbitone in preventing the recurrence of febrile convulsions. The children were randomly assigned to receive placebo or phenobarbitone. Follow-up visits were at one, four, eight and 12 months after the start of treatment. At each of these visits plasma concentrations of phenobarbitone were obtained (though withheld from parents and investigators until the end of the study), and parents were asked systematically about side-effects. After either eight or 12 months of treatment, a psychological test was administered to the child, according to age.

23 per cent of the 30 children in the placebo group had some transient side-effects; 43 per cent of the 35 in the phenobarbitone group had side-effects, these being transient in 23 per cent, dose-related in 11 per cent, and unacceptable in 9 per cent. These effects were primarily sleep disturbances – the child waking in the night ready for play – and fussiness and irritability in the day. No child was hyperactive on either phenobarbitone or placebo. The groups did not differ in their mean IQ scores. However, children with higher serum phenobarbitone levels performed more poorly on memory concentration tasks in relation to their general level of performance. Also children tested after 12 months had significantly lower scores on general comprehension, in relation to their basic level of intellectual functioning, than children tested after only eight months on phenobarbitone.

ROSS, E.M., PECKHAM, C.S., WEST, P.B., and BUTLER, N.R. (1980) *British Medical Journal,* 280, 6209, 207–10.

Epilepsy in childhood: findings from the National Child Development Study

Among a sample of nearly 16,000 children, all those born in England, Scotland and Wales in the week in March 1958 (the National Child Development Study sample) 1043 (7 per cent) were reported by their parents or a school doctor as having had at least one fit, faint, or turn by the age of 11. Where there were indications that the child had suffered from epilepsy (e.g. recurrent seizures, treatment with anticonvulsants, EEG investigations) further details were sought from the child's GP, hospital consultant and other medical sources. Scrutiny of the records showed that 606 (58 per cent) of the children did not have epilepsy, but had had a single seizure, faint, temper tantrum, breath-holding spell or behaviour disorder. An additional 39, reported by doctors or consultants as having 'epilepsy' did not fit in with the study definition of epilepsy as 'recurrent paroxysmal disturbances of consciousness, sensations or movement, primarily cerebral in origin, unassociated with acute febrile episodes'. Among the 366 children with febrile convulsions who did not develop afebrile seizures by the age of 11, there was no excess of perinatal problems, and school attainment at 11 was similar to children who had never had seizures.

Sixty-four children (4 per 1000) had a clear-cut history of two or more spontaneous afebrile seizures by the age of 11 and were regarded as definitely having epilepsy. This is similar to the average prevalence found in eight cross-sectional studies carried out over the last 20 years in various countries on the 10- to 20-year-old population.

Thirty-five (65 per cent) of the epileptic children had only grand mal (tonic-clonic) seizures. Only one child had petit mal (typical absences) alone, and a further eight started with petit mal and then developed grand mal. Two children had temporal lobe (complex partial) seizures, with relatively mild problems of giddiness and transitory confusion. All but one of the children had been prescribed anticonvulsants. Phenobarbitone was prescribed to 58 (90 per cent) but 36 (56 per cent) had their treatment changed to phenytoin, usually because of the side-effects of phenobarbitone.

After exclusion of twins and those with gross congenital abnormalities, there was little evidence that perinatal factors were the cause of epilepsy. Among single births, maternal bleeding before 28 weeks was the only perinatal difficulty more common in pregnancies resulting in a child with epilepsy. Thirteen children had abnormalities compatible with secondary epilepsy (e.g. cerebral palsy, sequelae of bacterial meningitis, head injury).

Fifty-nine of the children with epilepsy were followed up to the age of 16. Thirteen of the 22 (59 per cent) at special school were still having fits in their 16th year, but only eight out of 37 (22 per cent) of those at ordinary schools. Epilepsy was the major handicap in four of those at special schools, and mental retardation was the main handicap in the rest. Only three of those at special schools could read newspapers or fill in forms. The average reading and maths scores at 16 of the children with epilepsy at ordinary schools were slightly, but not significantly, lower than those of the whole study population (see Ross and West, 1977, for educational attainment at 11).

This study indicates that prospects are very different for the children with epilepsy who manage to stay in ordinary schools, and those in special education, whose main problem is often not epilepsy. (See also pp. 33, 39.)

OKUMA, T. and KUMASHIRO, H. (1981) *Epilepsia,* 22, 35–53.

Natural history and progress of epilepsy: report of a multi-institutional study in Japan

A study on the prognosis of patients carried out in Japan on 1868 patients from 20 institutions; the outcome of seizures and social adjustment was examined at intervals of ten, five, and three years after the onset of the illness. The overall rate of remission was 58.3 per cent, and the rate of normal social adjustment 62.6 per cent. A number of factors associated with a good prognosis are listed. Factors that determine the prognosis of social adjustment were found to be almost the same as those for remission or control of seizures.

THOMPSON, P., HUPPERT, F.A., and TRIMBLE, M. (1981) *British Journal of Clinical Psychology,* 20, 3, 155–62.

Phenytoin and cognitive function: Effects on normal volunteers and implications for epilepsy

Eight adult non-epileptic students were given either phenytoin or a placebo every day for three weeks; the design of the study was double-blind, so that neither subjects nor experimenters knew which of them was being administered. Before and after treatment all subjects were given tests of memory, concentration, perceptual speed, decision making, visuo-motor response, and motor speed. Subjects were also asked to describe their moods. Out of 16 tests, the subjects' performance was significantly poorer on two tests of memory, one of concentration, two of decision-making speed, and one of motor speed. A significant number of subjects described themselves as feeling fatigued. The authors conclude that the possible detrimental effects of phenytoin are of considerable importance, and that other drugs should be considered when making a choice.

STEDMAN, J., VAN HEYNINGEN, R., and LINDSAY, J. (1982) *Early Child Development and Care*, 9, 1, 65–82.

Educational underachievement and epilepsy. A study of children from normal schools, admitted to a special hospital for epilepsy

108 children referred to the epilepsy centre of the Park Hospital, Oxford, were studied. They were aged 9 to 13, had IQs over 70, and were attending normal schools. All children completed the WISC intelligence test or its revised version. Schoolteachers administered tests in reading, spelling and arithmetic. For each of the tests the children were grouped according to the relation between their 'Attainment Age' and 'Chronological Age', group 1 being good average, group 2 low average, group 3 moderately retarded, and group 4 severely retarded.

The proportions in each group for reading attainment were respectively 33 per cent, 16 per cent, 19 per cent, and 31 per cent; for spelling, 20 per cent, 10 per cent, 17 per cent, and 50 per cent respectively; for arithmetic, 16 per cent, 6 per cent, 20 per cent, and 56 per cent. There was a clear correlation between intelligence and attainment. Boys were more retarded in reading than girls. Out of the whole group, only 15 per cent were making fairly satisfactory progress by not being more than a year behind their chronological age in any of the three subjects. Nearly half the children were more than two years behind in two out of the three subjects. It is recommended that there should be more communication between doctors and teachers, so that teachers realize which of their pupils are epileptic and more able than they seem, and devise special teaching programmes to meet their needs.

BOURGEOIS, B.F.D., PRENSKY, A.L., PALKES, H.S., TALENT, B.K., and BUSCH, S.G. (1983) *Annals of Neurology*, 14, 438–44.

Intelligence in epilepsy: a prospective study in children

To investigate the long-term course of epileptic children's intelligence and cognitive skills, 72 children in St Louis, USA, were given a wide range of psychological tests; first, just after their epilepsy was diagnosed, and then each year afterwards for four years (severely retarded children were excluded). At the time of the initial testing their 45 siblings were also tested. In this study only the progress of intelligence scores is reported. The children with epilepsy were also given a thorough examination and the frequency of their seizures assessed; and anticonvulsant drug levels were measured at the time of each follow-up.

On the initial intelligence testing the average score of the epileptic children was 99.7, which was six points lower than that of their siblings – not a significant difference. The children with symptomatic epilepsy had a lower mean IQ than children with idiopathic epilepsy, a difference probably caused by pre-existing handicaps rather than the effect of seizures or drugs. Over the four-year period the epileptic group as a whole showed no drop in average IQ; but there was a sub-group of eight children (11.1 per cent) which showed a persistent decline of ten points or more. When the characteristics of this group were studied, it was found that these children had a higher incidence of drug levels in the toxic range than the rest of the group. They also had more difficulty in controlling seizures, and had been younger when seizures started.

Further statistical analysis suggested that drug toxicity (especially of phenobarbitol) and early onset of seizures predicted an IQ decrease more definitely than other factors such as poor control of seizures or type of seizures. The findings suggest that total seizure control, especially in young children, should not be achieved at the price of repeated episodes of drug toxicity.

GOODRIDGE, D.M.G. and SHORVON, S.D. (1983) *British Medical Journal,* 287, 6393, 641–7.

Epileptic seizures in a population of 6000. 1. Demography, diagnosis and classification, and role of the hospital services. 2. Treatment and prognosis

A total of 122 patients with epilepsy were identified in a survey of 6000 persons from a single general practice. 5.3 per thousand had active epilepsy. Overall patient assessment and monitoring was found to be poor; specialized epilepsy clinics are recommended. Recurrence after a first attack was found in four-fifths of patients, but generally the total number of seizures suffered by each patient was small, the period of active epilepsy short, and remission when it occurred was usually permanent. It is clear that the view that epilepsy is a chronic condition with a continuing liability to relapse is true for only certain cases, and this opinion reflects the selection bias of studies based on hospitals or institutions.

KURTZ, Z. (1983) In: ROSE, F.C. (Ed) *Research Progress in Epilepsy.* London: Pitman.

Special schooling for children with epilepsy

A study of all children attending six residential special schools for epilepsy. The children were multiply handicapped; only 5.6 per cent had no handicap beyond epilepsy, and 65.6 per cent had at least two more. The commonest additional handicaps were behaviour disorder and mental retardation. For 39 per cent, the chief cause for referral to a residential school was breakdown in their home situation. There was a higher than average percentage of single-parent families in the children's backgrounds, and a higher than average number of siblings in care. For 60 per cent of the children, problems such as financial difficulty, marital disharmony, parental ill-health and bad housing were recorded. Only 25 per cent had had full medical and educational assessment before being placed. Compared to earlier years, children were being placed at an older age (half of them at 13 or older), and were staying longer. The proportion going on to further education or training at 16 was 40 per cent. A follow-up showed that 30 per cent were in residential care after leaving, 24 per cent were employed, 19 per cent were at a training centre, and 21 per cent at home. It is recommended that the children should be under the care of a paediatric neurologist in a regional specialist centre working closely with other professionals; and that long-term support should be given to the child's family.

TRIMBLE, M.R. and THOMPSON, P.J. (1983) In: ROSE, F.C. (Ed) *Research Progress in Epilepsy*. London: Pitman.

The influence of anticonvulsant drugs on cognitive function and behaviour

A report of four investigations. In the first, the mean serum levels of anticonvulsant drugs in 312 epileptic children at a hospital school were studied, and related to their IQs. It was found that high levels of phenytoin and primidone were associated with a fall in IQ. Next, the effects of phenytoin, carbamazepine and sodium valproate were measured on non-epileptic volunteers, who were given tests of memory and recognition. Phenytoin – but not the other two drugs – impaired the subjects' performance slightly on the tests. Thirdly, the effects of drugs on behaviour problems in epileptic children were examined, and a non-significant association between antisocial behaviour and phenobarbitone was found. Finally, a 'Mood Adjective Check List' was used on the non-epileptic volunteers of Study 2; subjects reported a feeling of tiredness with phenytoin, but no effects from the other two drugs.

SECTION IV

Family Adjustment

The effects of a child's handicap on the family circle are difficult to research, and the studies on epileptic children's families are a mixed bag with mixed conclusions. In general, they point to understandable difficulties and distress for many parents.

The most detailed study, that of Ward and Bower (1978), contains a great deal of interesting anecdotal material. The general picture is of families coping adequately with inevitable problems. Ward and Bower found that parents continued to be shocked by fits, even when they had seen them often, and argue that the best help that can be offered is in controlling the seizures effectively. About half the parents who were interviewed had told friends and neighbours about the illness, usually without encountering prejudice (although people were often anxious about inviting epileptic children for fear of not being able to handle fits). Most children had not been told outright that they had epilepsy. In general, it was pre-existing family tension which affected the children, rather than the children's handicap affecting family tension, a finding supported by Goldin *et al.*'s (1971) study. (Hoare (1984), however, found a high proportion of the siblings of children with long-standing epilepsy to be psychiatrically disturbed themselves, possibly as a result of their sib's handicap.) Goldin and his colleagues also found, like Ward and Bower, that continuing uncontrolled seizures were particularly associated with distress within the family.

Two small-scale studies have attempted to assess interaction patterns within families with an epileptic child (Ritchie, 1981; Ferrari *et al.*, 1983). Ritchie found the families studied to be somewhat authoritarian, with the epileptic child rather left out; Ferrari and his colleagues found them to be less close than control families. These findings must be regarded as very tentative.

Tavriger's (1966) study touches on some of the fears and fantasies parents have about their children's epilepsy. As with other childhood handicaps, many parents feel an unjustified sense of guilt. It is clear from West's (1976) report on doctor–parent encounters that very often they need more explanation and support than they get. In a small sample of Dutch families, Mulder and Suurmeijer (1977) found parents uncertain about how much they should restrict the child with epilepsy and, again, anxious for more help. Voeller and Rothenberg (1973), Appolone, 1978 (see Section V, p.60), the British Epilepsy Association, 1981 (see Section V, p.62), and Ross, 1982a, 1982b (see Section V, p.63) spell out some of the factors that parents need to have explained, either by doctors or social workers. Ziegler's (1982) article stresses that professionals must learn to listen to what parents say (see Section V, p.64). The Report of the Working Group on Services for People with Epilepsy (1984) (see Section V, p.65) mentions in some detail the kind of support and information that might be provided.

TAVRIGER, R.
(1966)
Epilepsia, 7,
339–43.

Some parental theories about the causes of epilepsy

Parents of 118 epileptic children in London were noticed to produce many unrealistic explanations of the disorder in spontaneous discussions. These were divided into six groups. Group 1A covered ideas of epilepsy being caused by a single shock – for instance, father's desertion, being told of adoption. Group 1B covered various kinds of prolonged stress as cause. Group 2A covered physical trauma – falls, being slapped or shaken; Group 2B, physiological causes – digestion, delayed menstruation. Group 3 consisted of the one case where a genetic origin was wrongly blamed. Group 4 comprised miscellaneous explanations, such as 'punishment for sin'. The author suggests it may sometimes be helpful to parents to have such explanations to make sense of their distress.

GOLDIN, C.J.,
PERRY, S.L.,
MARGOLIN, R.J.,
STOTSKY, B.A.,
and FOSTER, J.C.
(1971)
Lexington, Mass.:
Heath Lexington
Books.

The Rehabilitation of the Young Epileptic; Dimensions and Dynamics

Subjects were 203 adolescents with epilepsy whose parents had responded to the questionnaire sent to them. Fifty-five out of the group had an additional disability. 26 per cent of the subjects had petit mal alone, 12 per cent grand mal, 6 per cent both petit mal and grand mal, 4 per cent psychomotor epilepsy and one Jacksonian epilepsy; of the rest, parents did not know what type of epilepsy the child had, or used incorrect names. The children with an additional disability were much more likely to have academic problems. Of the 167 still at school, 60 per cent were functioning at the appropriate level for their age; but 16 per cent of those without and 95 per cent of those with an additional disability were more than a year behind in grade, or in a special class.

Disagreement between the parents over child-rearing in such matters as protectiveness and discipline occurred in 35 per cent of the families. Three-quarters of the parents agreed that others should be told about the child's epilepsy; about 20 per cent agreed that it should *not* be disclosed, and 9 per cent were in disagreement over the issue. Two-thirds of the epileptic children got on well with their siblings, but more of those without (67 per cent) than of those with (43 per cent) an additional disability. Among the subjects with epilepsy alone, poor relationships with their siblings were related to early onset of epilepsy and to parent–parent or parent–child conflict. Almost 60 per cent of the parents placed no restrictions on the child because of his epilepsy, but the others restricted participation in sports or extended even stricter supervision. Two-thirds did not structure family activities around the child, and only 5 per cent said family activity was very restricted because of him.

More than two-thirds of the subjects interacted with other children in the area nearly every day, made friends easily, and showed no dislike of school, the two sub-groups not differing in these respects. Difficulty in making friends and dislike of school were related to seizures not being completely controlled and to conflict between parents. Dissatisfaction with the child's education was much more common among parents of children with an additional disability than it was among parents of children with epilepsy alone. Twice as many of the parents of children with an additional handicap said their children needed more planned recreational activities and other services such as professional counselling. Overall it is concluded that most of the problems of epileptic children with an additional disability come from that disability, while those of the child with epilepsy alone tend to come from family tensions rather than the epilepsy itself.

HARTLAGE, L.C. and GREEN, J.B. (1972) *Epilepsia,* 13, 21–6.

The relation of parental attitudes to academic and social achievement in epileptic children

In this study of 54 children with epilepsy, parental attitudes involving strictness, adherence to the parents' wishes, and 'treating the child as a person' were found to be positively related to the child's social maturity (Vineland Social Maturity Scale). Parental disapproval of activity by the child was negatively related to the child's academic achievement. Neither the type nor the frequency of seizures were related to social maturity. Average intelligence of the children, aged 6 to 16 and selected at random from the out-patient clinic of a large medical centre in the USA, was dull normal. Parental attitudes were measured by the Parental Attitudes Research Instrument.

VOELLER, K.K.S. and ROTHENBERG, M.B. (1973) *Pediatrics,* 51, 8, 1072–82.

Psychosocial aspects of the management of seizures in children

Based on work at an epilepsy centre in New York, the article urges that the feelings and fantasies of the whole family of the epileptic child must be taken seriously by helpers. The nature and causes of the disability must be made as clear as possible, especially to the child; misconceptions about EEG examinations clarified; parents helped with their painful feelings so that they can allow the child some freedom; and the question of correct medication followed up.

WEST, P. (1976) In: WADSWORTH, M. and ROBINSON, D. (Eds) *Studies in Everyday Medical Life*. Oxford: Martin Robertson, 13–31.

The physician and the management of childhood epilepsy

Using material from 64 observed doctor–parent encounters, the author examines the role of the doctor in the process by which a child who has had some kind of seizure becomes labelled as an 'epileptic'. There are differences in the definition of epilepsy; far from all children who have had seizures are classified as epileptic, and doctors are conscious of the stigma attached to the term. The doctor is also faced with uncertainties in determining the precise type of seizures and whether they will recur.

The first attendance at the hospital is crucial for the parents, who expect an explanation of the seizure and an account of what it signifies for the child. In the initial encounter the doctor maintains a tight control over the procedure, giving parents little chance to initiate discussion on what is concerning them, but often avoids specific diagnosis or discussion of the nature of the disorder and what it indicates for the child. However, in later encounters, as the parents become more experienced in coping with and evaluating the child's disorder they are more able to initiate discussion and 'force' the doctor to reveal information on diagnosis and prognosis, treatment and management. The uncertainty that arises from the parents' encounters with the doctor may cause them to turn to other, 'lay', sources of information, and sometimes to an alternative 'definition' of the situation, and to contravention of the doctor's rules on medication or participation in social activities.

MULDER, H.C. and SUURMEIJER, T.P.B.M. (1977) *Journal of Biosocial Science*, 9, 1, 13–24.

Families with a child with epilepsy: a sociological contribution

A pilot study of 13 epileptic children between 10 and 16 attending ordinary schools in the Netherlands. Long interviews were held, separately, with children and with parents. Half the parents said their freedom was curtailed by the child's epilepsy. Of the fathers, four were definitely rejecting. There was general uncertainty about how restrictive to be of the child's activities, and inadequate information from doctors. Most of the children were isolated from their peers, even after seizures had been controlled by medication, and were often teased at school. There was a tendency among them to feel stigmatized and to be over-dependent on parents

Of the 13 families, five were optimistic about the epileptic child's educational progress and the rest had doubts and reservations which seemed to be communicated to the child. Several parents blamed the sedative effects of the child's drugs for delayed school progress. There had been considerable delay in many cases in first seeking medical help; further delay could be caused by the general practitioner's referral to a specialist, notably in three cases. Further referral to a specialized epilepsy clinic was hit-and-miss and had usually been insisted on by the parents. Parents tended to be dissatisfied with the specialist's help and would have liked more time and attention. The authors emphasize that the sample was small and that results are tentative.

WARD, F. and BOWER, B.D. (1978) Supplement No. 39 to *Developmental Medicine and Child Neurology,* Vol. 20, No. 1.

A study of certain social aspects of epilepsy in childhood

A study of the impact on the parents of having a child with epilepsy. Interviews were unstructured, and carried out in the parents' homes by an experienced social worker. Seventy-eight mothers of 81 children with epilepsy were seen, and also 29 fathers. The children had attended a paediatric neurology clinic in Oxford. Children with major additional disabilities were excluded.

Of the many fears aroused by the child's epilepsy, that of the seizures themselves was dominant, being expressed by 70 per cent of the parents of the children whose epilepsy was newly diagnosed, and almost the same proportion (67 per cent) of parents of children whose epilepsy had been diagnosed earlier. Parents were anxious at having to cope, horrified by symptoms, and afraid of injury or even death for the child. Fears of mental abnormality were next commonest to fears of the seizures themselves, even when there was no evidence of it. Fears (expressed by a quarter of the parents) about heredity were not unrealistic, as a number of families had relatives affected, but they occurred even in families with no known history of epilepsy. Some parents (15) feared that a failure of care had precipitated the illness.

Relatives and friends: grandparents were usually told of the diagnosis and most had reacted with normal concern. But parents of 21 children thought that there had been excessive reactions by relatives, some being frightened of the seizures and of having to cope with them. Nearly half of the families had told friends and neighbours without experiencing any difficulties, some receiving support and sympathy. Generally the reactions of other children were quite good, the parents of only six children giving convincing evidence of teasing.

Schools: 50 of the 73 attended by the children appeared to the parents to be entirely accepting, some teachers being exceptionally understanding. Only two schools appeared to be predominantly rejecting, though in a few anxiety was shown, and expectations of underachievement. Only 15 children had been told that they had 'epilepsy' or 'fits', the majority (50) only being told enough to justify the medication, precautions over activities, and occasional visits to hospital. In 24 families there were disturbances which appeared to be related directly to the epilepsy, but in ten of these it seemed to be exacerbating pre-existing problems rather than being a prime factor, and in eight there were background factors which made the families vulnerable to stress. Sometimes, though, it does seem that the problems of severe illness can precipitate family problems.

Maladjustment: 22 of the 29 children who presented problems of management and adjustment had continuing seizures. In contrast, only ten of the 52 with no significant problems had continuing seizures, and in all but two they were now minor.

Identification of vulnerable families needs much time and care, and would probably be best achieved by a team approach, based on special centres for epilepsy. However, control of the seizures appears to be the key factor in satisfactory management of children with epilepsy – once these are banished other fears can be coped with, and adjustment made by the parents and the children themselves.

LONG, C.G. and MOORE, J.R. (1979) *Journal of Child Psychology and Psychiatry*, 20, 4, 299–312.

Parental expectations for their epileptic children

The study's aim was to compare parental attitudes and expectations for the epileptic child with those for a sibling. Nineteen families in Leicester were chosen with one epileptic child free of other disabilities and a sibling within two years of his or her age. Twelve of the sample had major fits, four had petit mal, three had both. On social class distribution there was an average spread. Kelly's repertory grid was used to elicit the ideas of the families about handicap, and 14 constructs defined ('expects to do well at school', 'expects to be moody', etc.). Factor analysis was used to define ideas of 'parent-in-relation-to-handicapped-child' and 'parent-in-relation-to-sibling'. A scale of social adaptation was completed by the mother for the children. The children completed self-esteem inventories, and did a test of reading ability.

On seven items of the grid there was a significant difference between expectations for the handicapped child and his or her sibling. Parents also saw themselves as more dominant and strict when dealing with the epileptic child. The majority thought that he or she should be supervised at all times: swimming, cycling, team games and climbing were prohibited in 28, 21, 16, and 11 per cent of cases respectively. More of the epileptics than of controls were described as socially isolated. Self-esteem scores were lower for the epileptics. On the reading test, 11 of the 14 epileptic children tested had a reading age below their chronological age, compared to six of their siblings. Parents' and teachers' ratings of psychiatric disturbance found the epileptic child to be more deviant than siblings. The authors conclude that parents can influence their children for the worse by their expectations, and that they need more information and advice.

RITCHIE, K.
(1981)
Journal of Child Psychology and Psychiatry, 22, 65–71.

Interaction in the families of epileptic children

From a centre in Australia, 15 families with an epileptic child and a well child and 15 matched control families were studied. A questionnaire was designed to obtain opinions on a variety of imaginary family situations, and in each case all four family members filled it in independently. Eight items were then chosen from the questionnaire on which there was disagreement. The family was brought together and asked to discuss the controversial items, and the discussion was recorded on video. The tapes were then watched by two independent judges and rated on a number of aspects such as 'problem-solving style'. When all the aspects were compared for the two groups of families, it was concluded that the families with an epileptic child acted as more efficient problem-solving units than the control families (disagreements and interruptions were minimized). Mothers in the epileptic group were more dominant than in the control families; also the epileptic children appeared to be rather withdrawn from family interaction. The findings are in general agreement with other studies of how families with a handicapped child cope; it is a style of interaction which may not be very helpful to the handicapped child.

FERRARI, M.,
MATHEWS, W.S.,
and BARABAS, G.
(1983)
Family Process, 22, 1, 53–59.

The family and the child with epilepsy

Forty-five children aged 6 to 12, and their families, were studied to discover what effects the ill child had on family functioning. They were divided into three groups of 15: epileptic children, diabetic children, and children without chronic illness. Several tests of adjustment and self-concept were administered at home to all the children and family members. The epileptic children were reported by parents to differ from the other two groups in a number of ways: they were more inclined to complain of rejection, to act in an immature way, to have periods of emotional distress, and to be aggressive towards the parents. Regarding the question of family cohesion, the families with an epileptic child reported themselves to be significantly less close than families in the other two groups. On the questionnaire measuring self-concept, the epileptic children showed a lower self-concept than the other two groups of children. It appears that there is a particular set of characteristics associated with epilepsy that distinguishes it from other chronic illnesses. One of these is the unpredictability of seizures. A larger-scale study is recommended. (See also p.23.)

HOARE, P.
(1984)
Developmental Medicine and Child Neurology, 26, 1, 14–19.

Psychiatric disturbance in the families of epileptic children

An examination of the extent of psychiatric disturbance in the parents and siblings of epileptic children. Twenty-nine children with newly diagnosed epilepsy and 29 with chronic epilepsy were used; the study group consisted of their parents, and their 46 school age siblings. For the parents, psychiatric disturbance was assessed by the 60-question General Health Questionnaire; for the siblings, the Rutter Parents' and Teachers' Scales were used. The siblings of the chronic epileptic group were significantly more disturbed than children in the general population. Siblings of the newly diagnosed epileptics were not significantly different from average, however. Parents of both epileptic groups were no more psychiatrically disturbed than average; but there was a significant association between disturbance in the epileptic child and disturbance in the mother. It is important that professionals are aware of the stressful effect of epilepsy on a family, and that doctors and schools maintain a close liaison.

SECTION V

General

Articles and books listed in this section cover a variety of background material which is apart from research: reports, review articles, general discussions, textbooks, and publications particularly for the lay public.

Central Health Services Council Advisory Committee on the Health and Welfare of Handicapped Persons (1969) Report of a Joint Sub-Committee of the Standing Medical Advisory Committee and the Advisory Committee on the Health and Welfare of Handicapped Persons (The Reid Report). London: HMSO.

People with Epilepsy

The committee was set up to consider health, welfare and other services jointly. It found that children with epilepsy were inadequately provided for medically and educationally, and were at a disadvantage socially. Two main recommendations were made: that the diagnosis, assessment, treatment and care of people with epilepsy should be provided by multi-disciplinary teams; and that a number of special centres should be set up for the comprehensive assessment and management of patients presenting particularly difficult problems.

Stores, G. (1971) *British Journal of Hospital Medicine,* 6, 207–14.

Cognitive functions in epilepsy

A review article of findings up to the date of publication. Subjects covered are cognitive function in temporal lobe epilepsy (including memory, learning, visual perception) and centrencephalic epilepsy; cognitive deficits in children; effects of anticonvulsive drugs; methods of re-educating children and adults.

Lindsay, J. (1972) *British Medical Journal,* 3, 283–5.

The difficult epileptic child

A description of the various specific difficulties experienced by the epileptic child – panic, rage, distractibility, learning difficulties. Careful and repeated assessments of the child, his or her family, and school, are called for if secondary and tertiary handicaps are to be reduced.

LIVINGSTON, S.
(1972)
Springfield, Illinois: Charles C. Thomas.

Comprehensive Management of Epilepsy in Infancy, Childhood and Adolescence

A detailed, comprehensive and clearly written account of all aspects of epilepsy, based primarily on the author's own studies of 20,000 epileptic patients, mainly children, seen at his epilepsy clinic. Clinical and electroencephalographic features of the main type of epilepsy are described. A major portion of the book is concerned with drug-management of the disorder. Other areas covered include surgical treatment of epilepsy, behaviour problems associated with epilepsy, and employment. The emphasis throughout is that the doctor should look at the 'whole child' and the problems that epilepsy creates for the child and his or her family, and not merely be concerned with the 'control' of seizures.

GASTAUT, H.
(1973)
Geneva: World Health Organization.

Dictionary of Epilepsy. Part I. Definitions

This dictionary, mainly covering terms related to the clinical aspects of epilepsy, presents an attempt to standardize the use of terminology. The opinions of experts from many countries have been taken into account in its preparation. It was originally prepared by Professor Gastaut, two further drafts being produced after WHO meetings in 1967 and 1968.

STORES, G.
(1975)
Developmental Medicine and Child Neurology, 17, 647–58.

Behavioural effects of anti-epileptic drugs

A review of the effects on mood and learning ability of the most widely used anticonvulsant drugs. The author argues that, while there is growing evidence that some of these drugs can have damaging effects, research methods have been crude and inadequate. More accurate observations, with different types of patient, are needed.

STORES, G.
(1976)
Public Health, 90, 4, 171–7.

The investigation and management of school children with epilepsy

A general discussion of the nature and problems of childhood epilepsy. Prevalence may be higher than is believed, because some forms of seizure are not recognized. Epilepsy in any case should not be referred to as if it were a disease entity in its own right, since it actually refers to a wide range of pathological states which have in common abnormal electrical discharge in the brain. Affected children appear to be particularly vulnerable from the educational and emotional point of view. Doctors and others involved in the care of these children need to learn more about the many aspects of seizure disorders, so that the children can be kept under careful supervision throughout their schooldays.

APPOLONE, C.
(1978)
Social Work in Health Care, 4, 2, 139–48.

Preventive social work intervention with families of children with epilepsy

A discussion of how social workers can help families with an epileptic child, illustrated with case histories. Parents need sensible and honest information to dispel their fears and fantasies. They need to be helped to set the right limits for the epileptic child without too much overprotection, and to tell neighbours or teachers of the problem without embarrassment.

DEPARTMENT OF EDUCATION AND SCIENCE
(1978)
Committee of enquiry into the education of handicapped children and young people (Chairman H.M. Warnock). London: HMSO (Cmnd. 7212).

Special educational needs: report of the Warnock Committee

The report of the Warnock Committee on the education of handicapped children and young people. Recommendations are made for the scope of special education, and for effective assessment and records during the school years. With an increasing number of children being placed in ordinary rather than special schools, teachers must be well informed, and specialist help available. Special attention is given to coordination of services, and to the appointment of an officer with responsibility for children with various special needs.

BRITISH EPILEPSY ASSOCIATION
(1978)

Epilepsy '78

First of a series of useful periodicals issued by the British Epilepsy Association. Papers were either commissioned by the association or collected from recent issues of journals. Fifteen papers cover many aspects of the disorder, starting from 'What is epilepsy?' and 'Who is epileptic?' to discussions of living with epilepsy, employment of epileptics, problems of travelling. More technical papers discuss sleep, trauma, serum drug levels, and the EEG.

British Epilepsy Association (1979)	**Epilepsy '79** Second in the British Epilepsy Association's series 'Perspectives on Epilepsy', written for both doctors and non-medical readers. It includes papers on schoolchildren, EEG assessment, 'kindling', drug treatment, temporal lobe epilepsy, with several chapters on some social problems of adults with epilepsy.
Betts, T.A. (1979) In: British Epilepsy Association, *Epilepsy '79.*	**Temporal lobe epilepsy** A useful and lucid explanation for the layman of this very complex subject.
O'Donohue, N.V. (1979) London: Butterworths.	**Epilepsies of Childhood** A comprehensive account of childhood epilepsies, dealing with emotional and educational problems, as well as describing different types of epilepsy and their management.
Trimble, M.R. (1979) Welwyn Garden City: Smith Kline French Laboratories Ltd.	**Neuropsychiatric Aspects of Epilepsy** A succinct account of the relationship between epilepsy and psychiatry – inter-ictal disturbances, personality disturbances, psychosis, drug treatment.
Laidlaw, M.V. and Laidlaw, J. (1980) Edinburgh: Churchill Livingstone.	**Epilepsy Explained** A brief, clear booklet written for those who have epilepsy and for their families, friends, teachers and workmates. There are five appendices which cover: the brain; driving licences; commonly used anti-epileptic drugs; addresses of associations for the epileptic; glossary.

PILLING, D.
(1980)
Unpublished manuscript.

The Child with Epilepsy: Research Review

An extensive research review carried out for the National Children's Bureau and available for consultation in the Bureau's library. A large number of research publications are summarized in detail and overall reviews of the findings given. The subjects covered include: definition and classification, intellectual and emotional development of the epileptic child, prevalence, aetiology, febrile convulsions, characteristics and prognosis of different types of epilepsy, and anticonvulsant treatment.

SUTHERLAND, J.M., TAIT, H. and EADIE, M.J.
(1980)
Edinburgh: Churchill Livingstone.

The Epilepsies. Modern Diagnosis and Treatment (3rd ed.)

Designed for medical students and doctors who deal only occasionally with epilepsy this is a useful, clearly written account of the nature and classification of epilepsy, the clinical features of the various types of epilepsy, the differentiation of epilepsy from other conditions with similar symptoms and the uses of various investigative techniques. The section on treatment includes an outline of the usage and side-effects of the anticonvulsant drugs in current use.

YOUNG, H.
(1980)
London: André Deutsch.

What Difference Does it Make, Danny?

A story for children, explaining the facts of epilepsy in simple and straightforward terms. Illustrated by Quentin Blake.

BRITISH EPILEPSY ASSOCIATION
(1981)

Epilepsy 80/1

Third in a series of the British Epilepsy Association's 'Perspectives on Epilepsy'. Articles include: stereotypes of epilepsy, psychosocial aspects, hysterical pseudoseizures, ambulatory EEG monitoring, drug prescribing, mental illness, group counselling, training of nurses.

BENIANS, R.
(1981)
Maternal and Child Health, December, 436–440.

Behaviour disorders in children associated with epilepsy

An overview of what fits feel like to children, and of how to manage both fits and behaviour problems of epileptic children and to counsel the adults concerned.

McMullin, G.P.
(1981)
London:
Duckworth.

Children Who Have Fits

A short and easy-to-read book specifically for parents. A brief list of suggested further reading is appended.

Reynolds, E.H.
and Trimble,
M.R. (Eds)
(1981)
Edinburgh:
Churchill
Livingstone.

Epilepsy and Psychiatry

An encyclopaedic review of the relation between the different forms of epilepsy and various types of psychiatric disturbance, both in children and adults.

Laidlaw, J. and
Richens, A.
(1982)
Edinburgh:
Churchill
Livingstone.

A Textbook of Epilepsy (2nd ed)

A collection of papers by specialists in various fields of epilepsy, written so that they present the latest understanding in that area to the intelligent non-medical person. Aspects covered include: the classification, symptoms and aetiology of fits in both adults and children; the EEG; psychological and social consequences of epilepsy; drug treatment; neurosurgery.

Ross, E.M.
(1982a)
Update, 1 March,
717–27.

Children's epilepsy – good doctoring really helps

For general practitioners, an outline of the forms of epilepsy that they may meet in their practices. Careful examination is urged; various types of anticonvulsant medication are listed and discussed. Schooling, activities and social problems are touched on.

Ross, E.M.
(1982b)
Health Visitor, 55,
1, 18–20.

Children with epilepsy: the health visitor's role

Outlines the different varieties of epilepsy, together with causes, prognosis, and prevention; advises on the sensible supervision of child and family.

Valman, H.B.
(1982)
British Medical
Journal, 284,
6325, 1321–2.

ABC of 1 to 7: Febrile convulsions

A useful brief summary of the symptoms, treatment and prognosis of febrile convulsions in young children.

ZIEGLER, R.G.
(1982)
Family Relations, 31, 3, 435–44.

Epilepsy: Individual illness, human predicament and family dilemma

The author points out that the family needs to find a way to deal with its helplessness and distress about the loss of control involved in epilepsy. There is a danger that it will not foster self-reliance in the child. The clinician must listen to the family's fears and preoccupations before attempting to advise. Illustrative case histories are given.

FENTON, G.W.
(1983)
In: ROSE, F.C. (Ed) *Research Progress in Epilepsy.* London: Pitman.

Epilepsy, personality and behaviour

An up-to-date review of the subject with a bibliography of 50 titles. Subjects discussed include the influence of temporal lobe dysfunction; classification of psychiatric disorders of epilepsy; personality and epilepsy; sexual dysfunction; epilepsy and violence; psychosis; causation of personality disorder.

MCGOVERN, S.
(1983)
London: Sheldon Press.

The Epilepsy Handbook (3rd ed)

A succinct introduction to epilepsy in children and adults. Chapters are included on schooling, family life, social provision, employment and medication. A glossary and a list of recommended reading are appended.

O'DONOHUE, N.V.
(1983)
Archives of Disease in Childhood, 58, 11, 934–7.

What should the child with epilepsy be allowed to do?

Swimming, bathing, sports, cycling and discotheques all carry some risk for the child with epilepsy. The author discusses the limits of what it is safe for the child to do, taking into account the severity and frequency of seizures.

ROSS, E.M., KURTZ, Z., and PECKHAM, C.S.
(1983)
Public Health (London), 97, 75–81.

Children with epilepsy: implications for the school health service

Recent research on epidemiology, diagnosis and management, and psychological and educational aspects of epilepsy is reviewed, and important recommendations for provision of services made. A multidisciplinary team headed by two paediatricians is recommended for each local health district, to be responsible for review of records, assessment, and liaison with general practitioners and school doctors.

CAMPION, J.
(1984)
Association for Child Psychology and Psychiatry News, 63, 14–18.

Behaviour problems in infant school children with convulsive disorder

An article for educational psychologists, with illustrative case histories.

WALLACE, S.J.
(1984)
Journal of Child Pychology and Psychiatry, 25, 1, 15–21.

Febrile convulsions: their significance for later intellectual development and behaviour

A review article assessing recent research. As well as intellectual development, other factors related to febrile convulsions are mentioned: behaviour problems, perinatal abnormalities, neurological status, parental management, anticonvulsants, and development of epilepsy. It is concluded that the results of early febrile convulsions are dependent on the pre-seizure status, unilaterality of the initial fit, recurrence of febrile seizures, continued neurological abnormalities, later progression to epilepsy, and socio-economic status. Febrile convulsions should be an indication that a neurodevelopmental examination is advisable.

WORKING GROUP ON SERVICES FOR PEOPLE WITH EPILEPSY
(1984)
London: HMSO.

Report to the Department of Health and Social Security, the Department of Education and Science and the Welsh Office.

The working group was set up to consider the recommendations of the Reid Report (see p.58), among other aims. It is concerned with provision of services for all people with epilepsy – hospital, primary health care and social services, and family support services; and a chapter is devoted to children with epilepsy. It is recommended that children with seizures should initially be assessed by a consultant paediatrician or paediatric neurologist, with the assistance of other staff where necessary. Following initial assessment the children should be cared for by the general practitioner or, for severe cases, a regional epilepsy clinic. The local education authority should be responsible for full assessment of special educational needs, if any, and for reviewing this assessment at least annually; inter-professional cooperation is essential for this to be effective. It may be necessary to provide either extra resources in an ordinary school, placement in a special unit attached to an ordinary school, or education in a special school. For children in ordinary schools, better support services will be needed, and the school health services must be kept fully informed by them. Teaching staff should also be kept informed, and school nurses could be of central importance. Special help and vocational counselling should be given at adolescence and in the early phase of education at college. For children with serious difficulties, there should be special assessment centres. If a residential school is necessary, efforts should be made to keep parents continuously involved, and close links should be established with special assessment centres.

Author Index

Laidlaw, J. and Richens, A. (1982) 63
Laidlaw, M.V. and Laidlaw, J. (1980) 61
Lewis, D.O., Pincus, J.H., Shanok, S.S. and Glaser, G.H. (1982) 22
Lindsay, J. (1972) 58
Lindsay, J., Ounsted, C. and Richards, P. (1979a) 20, (1979b) 20, (1979c) 21
Livingston, S. (1972) 59
Long, C.G. and Moore, J.R. (1979) 53
McGovern, S. (1983) 64
McMullin, G.P. (1981) 63
Mathews, W.S., Barabas, G. and Ferrari, M. (1982) 23
Mellor, D.H. and Lowitt, I. (1977) 38
Mellor, D.H., Lowitt, I. and Hall, D.J. (1974) 15
Mulder, H.C. and Suurmeijer, T.P.B.M. (1977) 51

Needham, W.E. *et al.* (1969) 31

O'Donohue, N.V. (1979) 61, (1983) 64
Okuma, T. and Kumashiro, H. (1981) 43

Pilling, D. (1980) 62

Özdirim, E., Renda, Y. and Epir, S. (1977) 38

Reynolds, E.H. and Trimble, M.R. (Eds) (1981) 63
Ritchie, K. (1981) 54
Ross, E.M. (1973) 33, (1974) 16, (1982a) 63, (1982b) 63
Ross, E.M. and Evans, D. (1972) 15
Ross, E.M., Kurtz, Z. and Peckham, C.S. (1983) 64
Ross, E.M., Peckham, C.S., West, P.B. and Butler, N.R. (1980) 41
Ross, E.M. and West, P.B. (1977) 39
Rutter, M., Graham, P. and Yule, W. (1970), 13, 32, 33
Ryan, R., Kempner, K. and Emlen, A.C. (1980) 8

Sands, H. and Zalkind, S.S. (1972) 5
Scott, D.F. (1978) 19
Sillinpaa, M. (1973) 34
Stedman, J., Van Heyningen, R. and Lindsay, J. (1982) 44
Stevens, J.R. and Hermann, B.P. (1981) 22
Stores, G. (1971) 58, (1973) 35, (1975) 59, (1976) 59, (1977) 18, 40, (1978) 19
Stores, G. and Hart, J. (1976) 37
Stores, G. and Piran, N. (1977) 18
Sutherland, J.M., Tait, H. and Eadie, M.J. (1980) 62

Tavriger, R. (1966) 49
Thompson, P., Huppert, F.A., and Trimble, M. (1981) 43
Trimble, M.R. (1979) 61
Trimble, M.R. and Thompson, P.J. (1983) 46
Tringo, J.L. (1970) 4

Valman, H.B. (1982) 63
Vinson, T. (1975) 6
Voeller, K.K.S. and Rothenberg, M.B. (1973) 50

Wallace, S.J. (1984) 65
Ward, F. and Bower, B.D. (1978) 52
West, P. (1976) 51
Whitman, S., Hermann, B.P., Black, R.B. and Chhabria, S. (1982) 23
Working Group on Services for People with Epilepsy (1984) 65

Young, H. (1980) 62

Ziegler, R.G. (1982) 64